Management of Aggressive Behavior

Crisis Prevention Intervention in Healthcare

JANE JOHN-NWANKWO RN, MSN

Management of Aggressive Behavior
Crisis Prevention Intervention in Healthcare

2*nd* Edition

Copyright © 2015 by Jane John-Nwankwo. RN, MSN

ISBN-13: 978-1514137475

ISBN-10: 151413747X

Printed in the United States of America.

www.djngbooks.org
www.janejohn-nwankwo.com
www.janejohn-nwankwo.org

Author's Audio books are available at audible.com

In Memory

In memory of my beloved late father John Chinyere Onwere, who taught me that I could do anything through Christ.

OTHER TITLES FROM THE SAME AUTHOR:

1. Director of Staff Development: The Nurse Educator (2nd Edition)
2. CNA Exam Prep: Nurse Assistant Practice Test Questions. Vol. One (2nd Edition)
3. CNA Exam Prep: Nurse Assistant Practice Test Questions. Vol. Two (2nd Edition)
4. IV Therapy & Blood Withdrawal Review Questions
5. Medical Assistant Test Preparation
6. EKG Test Prep
7. Phlebotomy Test Prep
8. The Home Health Aide Textbook (2nd Edition)
9. How to make a million in nursing 2015
10. Personality Types
11. How to Become a Better Wife
12. How to Become a Better Husband
13. How to Grow Your Small Business
14. It's in Your Hands: 5 Strategies to Achieving Your Life Dreams (Best Seller)
15. Weight Loss Inspiration

Simply search "Books by Jane John-Nwankwo" on Amazon!

www.djngbooks.org
www.janejohn-nwankwo.com
www.janejohn-nwankwo.org

Table of Contents

5

Preface

Having trained more than 1500 healthcare professionals on how to prevent crisis in the healthcare setting and how to professionally intervene in case it occurs, I decided to compile the ideas into a book.

-Author

Introduction

Crisis is a word used to define to a situation where assaultive behavior or violence has occurred. The essence of this book is to ensure that strategies are employed as early as possible in the process to prevent escalation of emotions that could result in assaultive behavior and crisis. Strength is giving to the old saying "Prevention is better than cure".

Jane John-Nwankwo CPT, DSD, RN, MSN, PHN

Chapter One

Outline

1. Introduction
2. Meaning of Crisis
   2.1. Definitions
   2.2. Background of Crisis
   2.3. Features of crisis
   2.4. Examples of Crisis
   2.5. Corresponding factors of assaultive behavior/ crisis
3. Types of crisis and their causes
   3.1. Criminal crisis
   3.2. Patient crisis
   3.3. Worker crisis
   3.4. Domestic crisis
   3.5. Verbal and physical crisis
4. Conclusion

Crisis prevention and Intervention in healthcare

1. Introduction.

The management of assaultive behavior is an effort to provide protection for the client and healthcare professional against any type of assault from either party. Assaultive behavior in the healthcare setting compromises the safety of the healthcare workers, the patients and visitors to the emergency rooms, mental health units, group homes, long term care facilities, etc. The abusive behavior undermines the efforts of the health care professionals that are in many cases, the victims. Poor behavior management costs the hospital time, money and high turnover rates. This chapter will discuss the meaning of assaultive behavior and crisis, as well as discuss the types and causes of crisis.

2. What is Crisis?

2.1. Definitions.

The meaning of crisis can be expanded by defining crisis, assaultive behavior and violence. According to Aguilera (1998, p. 12), crisis occurs when a person is unable to deal with problems that seem not to have a way out. The unresolved problems give way to anger, emotional unrest, tension, anxiety and stagnation.

Chou et al (2001, p. 139) points out that, assaultive behavior happens if the problem becomes persistent. The issues facing the individual become intolerable because the coping methods and accessible resources are inadequate. Crisis is viewed as a psychological instability that result from extreme situation or condition where the resolution is not attainable by means of common remedies. Crisis is a word used to define to a situation where assaultive behavior or violence has occurred. Great emphasis is placed on ensuring that strategies are employed as early as possible in the process to prevent escalation of emotions that could result in assaultive behavior and crisis.

Crisis is used to refer to assaultive behavior when it is extremely negative, unpredictable, uncontrollable and unacceptable in the society. Assaultive behavior involves an opportunity that the person in crisis uses to inflict injury or abuse another as Chou et al (2001, p. 139) mention. Violence is defined as the use of physical force with a motive to inflict injury. It is destructive, turbulent and forceful. Violence causes confusion and reveals accumulation of anger (Richter & Whittington 2006, p. 2). The word crisis, violence and assaultive behavior are often times, used interchangeably.

2.2. Background of Crisis.

Assaultive behavior can occur anywhere including the hospital. Medical departments have incidents that tantamount to assaultive behavior.

The incidents of assaultive behavior in medical departments are on the increase and need to be addressed. Crisis in the form of verbal abuse and physical abuse have occurred in different departments. The waiting area, mental health units and emergency departments are common areas where abuse can occur as Salmon and Varela (2007, p. 3) state.

People without any history of assaultive behavior or psychiatric condition can suddenly become combative. Assaultive behavior can be as a result of medical conditions or illnesses as well as certain medications. People of all ages can become assaultive. Assaultive behavior is present in people of all cultures, and socio-economic status. Crisis may also be as a result of unresolved emotional issues. People experiencing crisis desire to solve the problem as quickly as possible. They are influenced by actions or words from others, because they crave for a solution that can change their situation.

Assaultive behavior may be directed to relatives or family members, neighbors, roommates, authority figures, men, women, medical professionals, peers, bystanders and passive peers.

The assault can be done in the home, care facility, homeless shelter, hospital, school or correctional institutions. The common assaults involve the use of a weapon, physical violence and throwing of objects. Research shows that assaultive behavior is stimulated by anger, intimidation towards others, reaction to treatment, poor control of impulse, paranoia, and substance use, stimulation by auditory hallucinations

11

and money gain or stealing (Shaver and Mikulincer 2010, p. 54).

The medical conditions that have been found capable of leading to assaultive behavior include: vascular dementia, Alzheimer's, diabetes, stroke, delirium, excessive alcohol and medicine intoxication. Aggressive behavior has been found to emanate from patients with anxiety, irritability and following a stressful situation. Life threatening and altering situations have also been found to trigger aggressive behavior. Some clients have encountered crisis after having disabilities (Duxbury and Whittington 2005, p. 471).

In an attempt to deal with assaultive behavior in hospital departments, color codes are frequently used to define the kind of assault. Facilities choose colors like green or gray to mean an assaultive by a person without a weapon; silver to mean someone with a weapon, color blue means there is a medical emergency whereas code yellow means there is a bomb threat.

Features of crisis.

The meaning of crisis can be explained by discussing the characteristics or features which reveal the nature of crisis as Quanbeck (2007, p. 522) stipulates. Crisis that involves assaultive behavior or violence poses a threat.

The crisis reveals a persistent inability to change condition or eliminate the effects of the underlying issues. Crisis invites tension, confusion and fear. The person in crisis experiences a lot of discomfort. The person in crisis remains in a disequilibrium state.

Assaultive behavior or crisis portrays frustration, discrimination and antagonism. Precautions should be taken if the following signs are witnessed: a record of violence, violent expression, violent threats, intolerance and unmanageable anger. Healthcare professionals should take every statement made by mental health patients seriuosly. An example is a mental health patient that continually told his nurse that she reminded him of his mother. The healthcare professional at first took it as a complement, but as he continued to repeat it every shift he saw her on duty, she decided to check his history. To her uttermost shock, she discovered that the mental health patient hated his mother so much that he killed her. This discovery made her to initiate protective measures that ensured her safety until the patient was discharged.

Crisis can be said to be forthcoming if the client has a record of violent behavior and tendencies of verbal abuse towards others. Actions such as bullying, cruelty to animals, lighting fires, general defiance of rules and disrespect to socially acceptable behavior signify impending crisis. The person may engage in excessive lying, robbing and covert behaviors.

Crisis can be recognized from works of art such as painting and writing. People can write, paint, and compose poems or songs that express their intentions. Their thoughts can be revealed when they express their feelings. The expression is deemed to be a sign of assaultive behavior if the theme is against a specific person or comes from same origin without clear intentions. When the negative theme is persistent over a long period, it could result in crisis.

Constant threats from the same origin towards a specific person constitute abusive behavior. The threat made out of anger, hostility or disappointment, where the description of how the threat has been executed may become a crisis. The threat is well calculated before it is issued.

Intolerance, attitude motivated by beliefs, religion, mental abilities, sexual orientation, culture, ethnicity, and physical capabilities can signify crisis. The prejudice is revealed in the form of inability to cope with diversity. Unmanageable anger is a precipitate for crisis because it motivates aggressive behavior. When anger strikes, there is irritation, intimidation or bullying. Anger can lead to unexpected violence.

2.3.Examples of Crisis.

Crisis occurs when a person is physically sick or a close person is sick. Verbal abuse, insults, self-injury, throwing of objects, breaking and destroying objects, biting and pushing are examples of behavioral crisis. Other examples of crisis include: divorce or separation, loss of a person through death, accident, natural calamity, financial constraints, unwanted pregnancy and unemployment. If crisis is not intervened, it may lead to trauma.

2.4. Corresponding factors of assaultive behavior/ crisis.

In an attempt to understand the meaning of crisis, Aguilera (1998, p. 13) discussed three corresponding factors that a person with assaultive behavior experiences. The corresponding factors involves: perception, support and survival. Perception deals with the attitude and view the person with assaultive behavior has towards the underlying problem. The underlying problem could be finances, health, reputation, work, education and career which are very important to the person.

In a mental health patient, the individual has the paranoia that the nurses have bad plans against him. That is why, when there are a group of people around them, they need proper explanation as to why they are in the midst of a crowd.

If a good explanation is not proffered and on time, they may perceive themselves as 'trapped' and start violent actions like attacking anybody in the group or throwing objects.

15

Healthcare professionals must remember that mental health patients have auditory hallucinations which they feel compelled to obey. The next factor is the support that the assaultive person can get from people who are close to them. The person in crisis needs to have trust in a friend or family. The friend or family will give relevant assistance when required. The other balancing factor is the ability to find survival means. The individual's ability to cope with stress, anxiety and problems affects the response to crisis. The patients cope by doing exercise, denial, reasoning, taking medication and sleeping. When disequilibrium of the corresponding factors occurs, the person with the assaultive instinct can be said to be in crisis.

3. Types of crisis and their causes.

According to Colling and York (2010, p. 484) crisis can be distinguished according to the person who performs the assault and event. The four types of crisis include; criminal, patient, worker and domestic.

3.1. Criminal crisis/assaultive behavior.

The individual performing the assault is not related to the healthcare institution or the patient. This can be a person who commits a criminal act in the healthcare facility. They may rob or steal items belonging to patients, visitors or the health care facility. Criminal crisis happens because of availability of weapons such as guns.

When the hospital security is weak, the criminals may find the hospital accessible and commit crimes. The hospital may lack movement restrictions within the medical facility. The police have used the hospitals when holding criminals, who may take advantage of the situation and commit crime. Criminals are aware that hospitals have certain drugs that are controlled. The pharmacies or hospitals become a target for the criminals. The hospitals collect money from patients; the money becomes a target for robbery. Some criminals choose to abduct patients while they receive treatment and become violent when committing the act. Criminals causing abuse in hospitals consist of terrorists and unwanted visitors. The criminals pose as legitimate visitors to the patient or as health care workers (Salmon and Varela, 2007, p. 4).

3.2.Patient crisis.

The patient receiving healthcare service commits the act of aggression. Patient crisis is caused by patients who are receiving treatment. Some of the patients may be mentally disturbed and cause harm to others. Some patients who are mentally ill, abuse drugs, are traumatized or are frustrated by the situations; hence they become aggressive.

The patient may take advantage of a situation where the healthcare worker is alone in the health care facility. The health care worker may be giving an examination in an isolated room without the company of another person.

17

The patient may become aggressive if they are not attended to after a long time, owing to long periods of wait time.

The services being provided may become a cause of aggression. The patient may complain to get better services. Departments dealing with emergency, intensive care and head injury may have the highest cases of violence. The patient may attack the health care worker or another patient without warning. Patients with abusive behavior may take the form of verbal or physical abuse. They may use their nails, fists, body fluids, feet, teeth, food utensils, head, furniture or medical equipment to inflict injury on the healthcare professional (Charney and Fragala 2000, p. 163).

3.3.Worker crisis.

Worker crisis involves a healthcare professional of the healthcare facility. The aggression may be directed to another worker, patient or a visitor. Healthcare workers may have underlying disputes with each other that could result in aggressiveness. Depending on the nature of their dispute and anger management, the unresolved conflict may result in violence. The employees may work within the same department and rank at the same level. Other disputes may be between a healthcare worker and their supervisor.

The common forms of abuse can be overt or covert. Overt abuse can be in the form of verbal abuse.

Covert abuse takes the form of psychological harassment. The crisis may be motivated by the workers withholding information from each other, change of duties without consenting and informing the other, criticism, isolation and refusing to assist at work (Richter and Whittington 2006, p. 3). A typical example is a nurse who always comes late. Everybody on the unit knows that if they are assigned to relieve someone, the outgoing nurse would never leave on time. Such behaviors can result in unpleasant open confrontations and arguments on the medical unit.

Lannza (2006, p. 86) adds that, the health care worker may experience stress because of understaffing and workload. An example is when a nurse has patients of high acuity, most of them requiring special attention from her; She may lose control and start yelling to a nurse assistant for having not completed the vital signs yet. The nurse assistant, in turn may respond to her yelling using abusive words because she is also under stress, herself. Understaffing or work overload is a very common cause of crisis. Another cause of worker crisis is if the healthcare worker does not have any training to recognize and manage assaultive behavior. This book is being written to provide such training.

3.4. Domestic crisis.

Domestic violence occurs in the healthcare institution where the patient, the health care worker, relatives and friends to the patient engage in assaultive behavior.

19

The relatives and friend to the patient and friend may become impatient if the hospital takes long to attend to the patient, delays treatment or medical procedures. On another note, the relatives or friends may have personal differences with the patient and resolve them in the hospital.

The patient's relatives could become assaultive because of experiencing stress that comes with the patient illness. An argument can quickly escalate into a fight because of financial, emotional and excessive anger that either the patient or their visitor may be experiencing.

3.5. Verbal and physical crisis.

Physical abuse is directed to others, self and objects. The patient, health care worker, visitor or criminal may become violent to another person and bit, bite, slap, hit or push them. The patient can hurt self by biting, cutting and inflicting injury on the body. In some cases, a patient, visitor, health care worker or criminal may throw objects towards another out of anger. Another form of physical crisis is sexual abuse. Aggressive behavior towards objects results in damaged property.

Whether verbally or physically assaultive, a patient can become uncomfortable in their environment and become irritable as Duxbury and Whittington (2005, p. 472) discuss. A restrictive environment can become a source of conflict.

Patients who feel they are not listened to or treated accordingly can become abusive.

Inadequate communication between the patient and the healthcare worker can be the cause of aggression. The importance of *listening* to a patient cannot be overemphasized. Lending attentive ears to patients not only calms their fears and anxiety, but instills confidence in them that the healthcare team cares about them.

Crisis can be caused by internal, external or interactional factors. The patient may have mental illness or be under the influence of medication that can cause aggression. The healthcare worker or the patient's visitor may also have internal perception of the issues concerned and become violent. Internal aspects of crisis involve thought disorders, alcohol abuse and substance abuse.

External factors that emanate from the environment can trigger anger and violence. The patient can perceive the health care workers as the cause of their challenge and not being willing to assist. The healthcare workers may see the hospital structure and condition of work as dissatisfactory and become offended and hostile.

Patients need to feel secure and confident with the care they receive in a hospital. If a patient feels insecure, their privacy is intruded or they do not have quality services, they may become angry. Patients who have been disappointed with disrespect and unfriendliness when being given medication and meals have become resultantly aggressive.

21

Discomfort such as noise and extreme weather conditions trigger distress. Lack of freedom and rejection of examination or service in the hospital can cause irritation and violence. One of the hospital units that has the highest violence rates is the mental health unit owing to the fact that the behavioral health unit is a locked unit. Human beings like freedom and any situation that affects freedom triggers aggression even in mentally stable individuals.

Interactional factors refer to the situations that cause tension and abusive behavior. Lack of communication between the patient and health care worker or the relative can cause aggressive behavior. Failure to listen and to be considerate contributes to disappointment that could lead to abusive behavior. Disagreement and poor relationship between the patient and the healthcare worker can stimulate conflicts that cause aggression. The healthcare worker may lose patience because of the health facility's pressure to work in a challenging environment.

4. Conclusion.

Crisis refers to assaultive behavior or violence that occurs after an individual in unable to change uncomfortable circumstances, becomes unpredictable, unmanageable and their behavior is not approved in the society. Crisis happens when an individual cannot change circumstances and the available resources are limited.

Types of crisis/ assaultive behavior include: criminal, patient, worker and domestic crisis. People with crisis engage in physical and verbal abuse. Crisis is triggered by internal, external and situational factors. Medication, illness, substance abuse, lack of training for workers, unresolved emotional issues, lack of communication, long waiting time, delayed or denied services and poor security could lead to assaultive behavior.

References

Aguilera, D. C. (1998). *Crisis intervention: Theory and methodology* (8th ed.).

St. Louis: Mosby

Charney, W., and Fragala, G. (2000). *The Epidemic of Health Care Worker Injury: An Epidemiology.* Florida: CRC Press.

Chou, K. R., Lu, R. B., and Chang, M. (2001). Assaultive behavior by psychiatric in-patient and its related factors. *Journal of Nursing Research,* 9 (15), 139- 151.

Colling, R. L., and York, T. W. (2010). *Hospital and healthcare security* (5th ed.). New York: Elsevier Inc.

Duxbury, J., and Whittington, R. (2005). Causes and

management of patient aggression and violence:

staff and patient perspectives *Journal of Advanced*

Nursing 50(5), 469–478.

Lannza, M. L., Zeiss, R and Rierdan, J. (2006).

Violence against psychiatric nursing. *Contemporary*

Nurse, 21(1), 85-93.

Quanbeck, C. D. (2007). Categorization of aggressive

behavior acts committed by a chronically

assaultive state hospital patient. *Psychiatric*

Services 58 (4), 521- 528.

Richter, D., and Whittington, R. (2006). *Violence in*

Mental Health Settings: Causes, Consequences,

Management, Berlin: Springer.

Salmon, N., and Varela, R. (2007) *Learning to manage*

assaultive behavior. New York: AMN Healthcare

Services Inc.

Shaver, P. R., and Mikulincer, M. (2010) *Human Aggression and Violence: Causes, Manifestations, and Consequences*. Washington: American Psychological Association.

Crisis Intervention and Prevention in Healthcare
Questions Chapter 1

1. _____ behavior involves an opportunity that the person in crisis uses to inflict injury or abuse another

   A. Combative

   B. Rude

   C. Assaultive

2. What is defined as the use of physical force with a motive to inflict injury

   A. Violence

   B. Conflict

   C. Escalation

3. Which of the following causes confusion and reveals accumulation of anger

   A. Conflict

   B. Violence

   C. Assaultive

4. The word crisis, violence and assaultive behavior are often used interchangeably

   A. True

   B. False

C. None of the above

5. Research shows that assaultive behavior is not stimulated by anger and intimidation towards others

   A. True

   B. False

   C. None of the above

6. All of the following include medical conditions that are capable of leading to assaultive behavior except

   A. Cancer

   B. Diabetes

   C. Stroke

7. Life threatening and altering situations have also been found to trigger aggressive behavior

   A. True

   B. False

   C. None of the above

8. Which of the following is precautions taken for assaultive behavior

   A. Violent threats

   B. Intolerance

C. Both a and b

9. Healthcare professionals should not take every statement made by mental health patients seriously

   A. True

   B. False

   C. Neither a or b

10. Crisis is viewed as a _____ instability that result from extrme situation

    A. Psychosocial

    B. Physiological

    C. Psychological

11. _____ is the word used to define to a situation where assaultive behavior or violence has occurred

    A. Crisis

    B. Conflict

    C. Violence

12. Assaultive behavior may be directed towards which of the following

    A. Passive peers

    B. Roommates

    C. Family members

D. All of the above

13. The colors use by hospital department to mean an assaultive person without a weapon is

    A. Silver

    B. Green or gray

    C. Blue

14. Crisis cannot be recognized from work of art such as painting and writing

    A. True

    B. False

    C. None of the above

15. _____ deals with the attitude and view the person with assaultive behavior has towards the underlying problem

    A. Support

    B. Survival

    C. Perception

16. Mental health patients have auditory hallucinations which they feel compelled to obey

    A. True

    B. False

C. None of the above

17. Criminals are aware that hospitals have certain drugs that are controlled and money

    A. True

    B. False

    C. None of the above

18. Which of the following is common causes of crisis

    A. Loving family

    B. Correct staffing

    C. Understaffing or work overload

19. Crisis can be caused by internal, external or interactional factors

    A. True

    B. False

    C. None of the above

20. Lack of _____ between the patient and health care worker or relative can cuse aggressive behavior

    A. Contact

    B. Communication

    C. comfort

Chapter Two

Outline

1. **Introduction**

2. **General safety measures for the healthcare professionals**

2.1. Administration and healthcare professional support

2.2. Environmental analysis

2.3. Risk reduction

2.4. Training

2.5. Regular review

3. **Personal safety measures**

3.1. Education and training

3.2. Self defense mechanisms

3.3. Ways of de-escalating violence

3.4. Be alert

3.5. Self-care for professional healthcare

4. **Conclusion**

Safety Measures to prevent or reduce crisis in healthcare

1. Introduction.

The management of assaultive behavior in healthcare facility requires enhancing the safety of patients, healthcare professionals and visitors. This chapter will discuss general and personal safety measures in the healthcare facility.

2. General safety measures for the healthcare professionals.

General safety measures for health care professionals facilitate sustenance of a good working environment and prevention of assaultive behavior. The safety measures should be adjusted according to specific conditions or nature of environment that healthcare professionals work in. General safety measures consist of five elements; administration and healthcare professional support, environmental analysis, risk reduction, training and regular review (Occupational Safety and Health Administration, 2011, p. 14).

2.1. Administration and healthcare professional support.

The healthcare administration and the facility employees must engage in safety plans. The plans involve appointing teams of healthcare workers, employers, committees and representatives of the safety plans. The healthcare professionals who are expertise in crisis management should be involved.

33

The representation should be fair in terms of departments and shifts. Drills should be conducted for workers in the different shifts. i.e. drills should be conducted for the night shift workers, morning shift workers and mid-shift workers, so that everyone is equipped with knowledge of early recognition and appropriate intervention of assaultive behaviors. Tasks should be allocated to the different stakeholders who may include: employer's representative, healthcare professionals, security representatives and administrators. Healthcare professionals able to deal with head injury, substance abuse, psychiatry and dementia should be advised to assist when the need arises. A working structure and applicable policies can be designed. The policies should represent diverse needs of the departments and provide procedures to be used in case of crisis.

The safety plan should take into consideration the physical, psychological and emotional safety and health of the healthcare professionals.

A balance between the safety and health needs of the healthcare professional, patient or visitor should be recommended. Representatives, experts, committees and teams with assigned tasks or responsibility should inquire and understand their responsibility in full detail.

After proper understanding, they can be authorized and be given resources that will enable them provide administration and support. Representatives, experts, committees and teams should demonstrate accountability.

In the case of assault and crisis, the involved parties can be given counseling and treatment. Those who have undergone assault can share their experiences. All the stakeholders can give their support in the enactment of the recommended policies.

The healthcare professionals ought to be committed to comply with the policies and give feedback. Suggestions on safety and complains should be given the appropriate authority. Cases of crisis should be reported in time and appropriately. The healthcare professionals should be willing to participate in teams, committees or as representatives in educational programs.

2.2.Environmental analysis.

Environmental analysis will consist of an assessment where potential risks are identified. Procedures, threats and factors that motivate crisis are pointed out. The analysis will take into consideration incidents and history of assaultive behavior in the same and other healthcare facilities. The information will be retrieved from compensation claims and patient records.

Environmental analysis in the workplace focuses on records, surveys and security details. The records will give details of occurrence of incidents in various departments, healthcare professionals by title, time, activities in progress and frequency of occurrence. The incidents are analyzed and compared with similar reports from other healthcare facilities. Surveys taken from healthcare professionals can be a source of information.

The surveys can assist in determining procedures that lead to risks, inadequate measures, inadequate resources, failures, policies and activities that need to be changed. Characteristics of those involved in the assaultive behavior and recommendations are considered. Risky procedures and locations should be identified. Some of the factors may involve physical conditions like the layout of the hospital facility. Isolated locations, lack of communication, security problems and inadequate light that contribute to risk.

2.3.Risk reduction.

Risk can be reduced by adopting measures, procedures and administrative work that will assist in preventing and controlling the occurrence of assaultive behavior in the health facility. The administration should make physical changes to the environment. The changes may consist of adequate lighting in dark rooms and increased space where necessary. There should be light both inside and outside the healthcare facility. Alarm system and panic buttons can be installed so that a potential victim can get assistance. The phones and radio systems should be working at all times and reliable.

The security should be enhanced by using metal detectors so that dangerous weapons such as knives and guns can be detected before they are smuggled into the healthcare facility. Places that are identified as high risk can be given video surveillance round the clock.

Curved mirrors can be placed in concealed locations and corridor intersections. Areas that are prone to risks include the triage, nurses' station, reception and admitting areas. Deep service counters, bullet proof counters and shatter proof glass can be used. A separate room can be used as a safe room when attending to emergencies. For patients who want to escape, high ceiling rooms can be provided. Rooms used for counseling should have alternative exits. Rooms used for treatment or counseling should be locked.

The waiting room should be made comfortable with chairs and reading materials. The furniture should be placed properly to avoid falls. The number of furniture in the consultation room and activity room should be limited. The furniture should not be fixed or possess sharp ends. Avoid placing vases, pictures or trays where they are visible or in high risk areas. The healthcare professionals will require different washrooms from the patients installed with locks. Broken furniture, bulbs, windows and locks should be replaced.

Thorough searching of mental health patients during admission must be done to prevent smuggling tiny weapons like razor blades, needles, tiny pocket knives, etc. Every pocket comb must be completely examined as some pocket combs, when unfolded are actually pocket knives. Patients must account for their tooth brushes as some mental health patients break their brushes and use them as weapons.

Policies should clearly state that assaultive behavior is not acceptable in the hospital. In the case of crisis, a report should be written and depending on the severity, the police can be involved. Advice should be given to healthcare professionals on the procedure of reporting and claim after a crisis. Train and place emergency teams where they can assist in the event of assaultive behaviors. Waiting time can be reduced and patients receive timely information while in the waiting room or undergoing a procedure. Visitors to patients should be restricted especially if there is a history of assault. Meals times should be observed and call lights treated as emergencies. Information on hospitalized patients should be restricted. Patients including psychiatric patients who are admitted should be supervised. Additionally, the pharmacy should be a controlled area (National Collaborating Centre for Nursing and Supportive Care, 2005, p. 1).

Bartholomew (2006, p. 23) adds that, healthcare professionals should be encouraged to work with partners where there is emergency or at night. When patient note that the unit is sufficiently staffed, they reduce their plans to assault. An evacuation plan should be designed and presented. Patients with assaultive behavior can treated in an open area. After an assaultive incidence the healthcare professionals should receive assistance.

2.4.Training.

Mason and Chandley (1999, p. 65) points out that training provides understanding on assaultive behavior, and enables the healthcare professionals to prevent and handle impending crisis appropriately. Training educates the healthcare professional on policies concerning assaultive behavior in the healthcare facility. Additionally, the healthcare professionals will be able to recognize risks, escalating behavior, warning signs, prevention methods and what to do in the case of a crisis. They will know where to report and how to report an unpleasant incident. Additional information about cultural diversity, personality differences and various ailments that contribute to assaultive behavior can be shared (Flannery 1998, p. 91). Moreover, they will know how to complain or itemize concerns, where to complain and how to get compensation. Training should be given to healthcare professionals, managers, supervisors and security workers.

2.5.Regular review.
Record of assaultive behavior should be made. The records should be analyzed to give information on risk factors and patterns of assault. An analysis will provide a basis for identifying gaps that can be made to manage assaultive behavior in the healthcare facility. Important items for record include; type of injury, number of injury, assault, threat, accidents, type of crisis, response to crisis, persons involved, identified problem and solutions. A regular evaluation should be conducted to identify areas that need change and check if policies are being observed.

3. Personal safety measures.
Healthcare professionals should assume responsibility for their individual safety.

39

Healthcare professionals need to protect self from aggressive behavior directed by patients, visitors and other healthcare professionals. This can be achieved through: education and training, self defense mechanisms, de-escalating violence, being alert and practicing extreme environmental awareness. On no account should the healthcare professional think that the psychiatric patient has adjusted to his medications and is no longer capable of assault. They must always be seen as manipulators. Sleeping on duty is one of the most dangerous mistakes when working on the mental health unit. Healthcare workers should take their breaks in protected rooms that the patients do not have access to. There was a case of a nurse on duty who was supposed to be watching a patient on a one-to-one observation to prevent suicide. Unfortunately, the nurse slept off, the patient beat the nurse so bad that by the time, the other workers could arrive, she was already unconscious. She was rushed to the emergency room and suffered paralysis from spinal cord injury inflicted by the patient.

3.1. Education and training.

Healthcare professionals can engage in ongoing training for their personal benefit as Linsley (2006, p. 32) recommends. The employee will assist in raising awareness of the environment, control in crisis and boost individual confidence.

Employees will learn safety places and techniques for conducting self at work.

Training will educate the healthcare professionals on the techniques for de-escalating violence.

Learning will enable the healthcare professionals recognize factors contributing to agitation and self-protection techniques. Bibby (1995, p. 56) found out that, education gives the healthcare professional ability to predict behavior and adjust to being neutral to diffuse anger. Likewise, communication skills such as listening and responding appropriately will be acquired. Talk slowly with a low calm and audible voice. The healthcare professionals should cooperate with the organization when asked to join in programs. The policies concerning the working environment should be followed. All incidents should be reported to the appropriate authority so that appropriate measures are made to prevent further assaultive incidents. The healthcare facility puts a lot of effort to prevent and manage crisis. Therefore, reporting to the risk management department facilitates development of appropriate strategies against assaultive behavior. Strategies will enable the professionals prevent possible violent attacks. Healthcare professionals should commit self to read and analyze reports carefully to facilitate early recognition of patients with aggressive behavior.

3.2.Self defense mechanisms.
        A professional healthcare worker can practice safety by adapting appropriated behavior and choosing to defend self in case of a physical assault.

41

When at risk, they can call for assistance, keep the way clear and escape if possible. Practice patience and encourage conversation. Avoid showing the aggressive person the back, try to choke them from the back and get away. Another way of protecting self is by chokeing the aggressor from the front if they attack from the front. If the attacker grabs the arm, try to push the arms downwards then twist towards the escape route.

Personal safety measures require a healthcare professional to avoid working in isolation where there are patients with assaultive behavior. Work where others can see you. Avoid entering where people with assaultive behavior can lock you inside. Always have access to the door, do not let your patient stand at the door while you are inside.

3.3.Ways of de-escalating violence.

For personal protection, a healthcare professional can bargain and apply conflict resolution when facing a crisis. Conversation should be conducted in a calm environment with the worker listening to the person in crisis. Confrontation should be avoided, keep away from persistent contact of the eyes. It is wise to stay away from interacting and request for audience. Showing empathy, understanding and showing concern to the assaultive person can reduce tension. Healthcare professionals can use moderate tone, calm voice and appropriate choice of words when communicating. Redirecting the topic can be another significant method of de-escalating assaultive behavior.

Refrain from responding to threats with other threats since it can activate violence. An example is an incident where a mental health patient told a nurse that she should be ashamed of herself because all she does is come to the hospital to give meds to make a living. The nurse replied her that she should be more ashamed that her teenage mates are in college, working, or at least doing something with their lives, but she is 'living' in the hospital. The patient reacted in a way that was very notable. When the root of the behavior was researched, the nurse gave the story. Avoid commanding and when given a chance acknowledge their feelings. Evade walking close, jumping, touching or moving closely to the person with signs of aggression. Avoid touching objects that could be perceived as a weapon.

Communicate when you want to move or touch them by making them understand. The healthcare professional can request for permission before dressing a wound, changing beddings, taking temperature or recording blood pressure, when conducting medical procedures (Scott et al 2001, p. 61).

3.4. Be alert.

The healthcare professional should be very alert, taking precaution when a threat of aggressiveness is imminent. They should enact a safety plan without delay if a patient is assaultive. If the healthcare professionals are threatened, they should avoid using suggestive body language and words that may reveal their feelings to the patient.

If the patients detect their feelings they may withhold information, feel threatened and react negatively to the healthcare professional's instructions (Hamilton 2011, p. 1).

According to Hughes (2008, p. 39), the healthcare professionals should be able to recognize risks and signs that can lead to aggressive behavior. Nurses and other healthcare workers should recognize signs of assaultive behavior. When a person shows frustration, anger and physical gestures depicting aggression, they can be viewed as a threat. Recognize patients with conditions that cause aggression such as mental illness and head injury. Keep a distance if the person with a sign of aggression is under the influence of drugs or alcohol and stay clear of things that could provoke them.

Remain alert at all times because every situation is unique and should be handled depending on the circumstances. Healthcare professionals should analyze the situation and type of occurrence before attending to the patient. Exercise vigilance when dealing with the patient.

If the person is capable of becoming violent, ask for company. Ensure there is an open exit, and be sure no object or patient is blocking the exit in case you might need it. The healthcare professional should call for help right away if they cannot exit.

Watch for objects that can be thrown or used as a weapon. Keep distances to avoid being hit on the head suppose the person in crisis holds an object. Stand away from the patient's fists.

44

The healthcare professional should not allow the person in crisis push them to a corner. Keep keys away from display. Keys should be hidden because they can provide access to other rooms or aid in escaping. In case the threat on the healthcare professional is persistent, it may be necessary to move their working station and request for security. A time off may be considered if the life of the healthcare worker is in danger.

3.5.Self-care for professional healthcare

Healthcare professionals may become busy and fail to take care of their needs which can contribute to emotional outbursts. With the knowledge of their working environment and challenges, healthcare workers should take care of their emotional, physical and psychological needs. The healthcare professionals should regulate the number of hours in a day so that they are not overworked.

After work they should rest and get enough sleep. It is very ironical how healthcare professionals preach so much about rest but rarely observe it. They are many a time ruled by the amount of money they will make when they work overtimes. Lack of time for oneself can predispose to lack of mental alertness when assaultive behavior is imminent. Evade situation that can cause burnout and fatigue. Healthcare professionals can manage stress by performing hypnosis techniques. The healthcare professionals should take a balanced diet and have regular physical exercises. They can maintain social relations with family and friends for social support.

Healthcare professionals should maintain their spiritual relations and stay proactive (National Collaborating Centre for Nursing and Supportive Care, 2005 p. 1). Their days-off should be enjoyed to the fullest so that they are mentally refreshed to return to work.

4. Conclusion.

General and personal safety measures facilitate prevention and intervention of aggressive behavior. General safety measures require the facility administration and healthcare professionals to collaborate in the development plan of policies and intervention of violent behavior. After developing a plan, the selected teams, commissioners and representatives analyze the environment to identify the risk factors. The healthcare facility together with professionals commit themselves to strategies that help in reducing risks that could contribute to crisis. Healthcare employees are trained on the safety measures, warning signs and intervention.

Once the plans are implemented, they are reviewed regularly and adjusted accordingly. General safety measures require improvement of the physical environment, improved working relations with patients and other healthcare employees, participation in implementation plan and reporting incidents correctly to the right authorities.

Personal safety measures encourage healthcare professionals to ensure they receive training and competence in assaultive behavior prevention and management.

They can protect themselves using ways of de-escalating violence and self defense mechanisms in cases of assault. Healthcare professionals should remain alert to signs of assaultive behavior as well as practice self care.

Reference

Bartholomew, K. (2006). *Ending Nurse-To-Nurse Hostility Why Nurses Eat Their Young and Each Other.* Danvers: HCPro.

Bibby, P. (1995). *Personal Safety for Health Care Workers (Suzy Lamplugh Trust)* Farnham: Ashgate Publishing Limited.

Flannery, R. (1998). *Violence in the Workplace Managing Assaultive Behavior.* New York: Crossroad publishing company.

Hamilton, P. M. (2011). *Psychiatric Emergencies: Caring for People in Crisis.* Wild Iris Medical Education Inc.

Hughes, R. (2008). Patient safety and quality: an evidence based Handbook for nurses. Agency for Healthcare Research & Quality.

Linsley, P. (2006). *Violence and Aggression in the Workplace: A Practical Guide for All Healthcare Staff.* Abingdon: Radcliffe Publishing.

Mason T & Chandley M. (1999). *Management of violence and aggression.* Philadelphia: Churchill Livingstone.

National Collaborating Centre for Nursing and Supportive Care. (2005)VIOLENCE: THE SHORT- TERM MANAGEMENT OF DISTURBED/VIOLENT BEHAVIOUR IN PSYCHIATRIC IN-PATIENT SETTINGS AND EMERGENCY DEPARTMENTS. London: National Institute for Clinical Excellence.

Occupational Safety and Health Administration (2011). *Guidelines for Preventing Workplace Violence for Health Care & Social Service Workers.* United States: U.S. Department of Labor.

Scott, S., Chris, W., and Sorensen, S. (2001) Essentials of aggression management in health care. New Jersey: Prentice Hall.

Crisis Intervention and Prevention in Healthcare
Questions Chapter 2

1. General safety measures consist of _____ elements

    A. Three

    B. Four

    C. Six

    D. Five

2. Drills should be conducted for workers in the different shifts

    A. True

    B. False

    C. B only

    D. None of the above

3. A balance between the safety and health needs of the healthcare professional, patient or visitor is not recommended

    A. True

    B. False

    C. None of the above

    D. All of the above

4. _____, experts, committees and teams should demonstrate accountability

   A. Telecommunications

   B. Organizations

   C. Representatives

   D. Doctors

5. Surveys taken from healthcare professionals can assist in determining which of the following

   A. Policies and activities

   B. Risks

   C. Failures

   D. All of the above

6. All of the following is included in risk reduction except

   A. Adequate lighting in dark rooms

   B. Alarm system is unnecessary

   C. Phone and radio systems should be working at all times

   D. None of the above

7. The pharmacy should be a controlled area

   A. True

B. False

C. None of the above

D. All of the above

8. Patients with assaultive behavior should be treated in an

    A. Closed area

    B. Secluded area

    C. Open area

    D. None of the above

9. Training educates the healthcare professional on policies concerning assaultive behavior in the healthcare facility

    A. True

    B. False

    C. Both a and b

    D. None of the above

10. Healthcare professionals should not assume responsibility for their individual safety

    A. True

    B. False

    C. A only

D. None of the above

11. Sleeping on the job is one of the most dangerous mistakes when working on the mental health unit

    A. True

    B. False

    C. All of the above

    D. None of the above

12. Which of the following are ways to defend yourself from a physical assault

    A. Always have access to the door

    B. Call for assistance

    C. Practice patience

    D. All of the above

13. One way of de-escalating violence is to avoid confrontation

    A. True

    B. False

    C. B only

    D. None of the above

14. Redirecting the topic is a significant method of de-escalating assaultive behavior

A. True

B. False

C. All of the above

D. None of the above

15. The healthcare professionals should regulate the number of hours in a day so that they are not overworked

A. True

B. False

C. All of the above

D. None of the above

16. Healthcare professionals should not take a balance diet and have regular physical exercise

A. True

B. False

C. None of the above

17. Causes of crisis should be reported in time and appropriately

A. True

B. False

C. None of the above

18. The number of furniture in the consultation room should be limited

    A. True

    B. False

    C. None of the above

19. Policies should clearly state that assaultive behavior is not acceptable in the hospital

    A. True

    B. False

    C. None of the above

20. Healthcare professionals should commit self to read and analyze reports carefully to recognize patients with aggressive behavior

    A. True

    B. False

    C. None of the above

Chapter Three

Outline

1. Introduction
2. The assault cycle
2.1. Trigger phase
2.2. Escalation phase
2.3. Crisis phase
2.4. Recovery phase
2.5. Post crisis phase
3. Aggression and violent predictive factors
3.1. Demography and personal history
3.2. Individual disorders, sickness and substance abuse factors
3.3. Situational factors
3.4. Actuarial and clinical predictive factors
3.5. Broset violence register
4. Conclusion

Crisis prevention and Intervention in healthcare

1. Introduction.

A number of healthcare professionals have experienced violence in the workplace. Violence has been exhibited by patients, workmates and visitors to the healthcare professionals. A clear pattern of how violence occurs has been identified. There are preceding observations that can be made before a person progresses to become assaultive (Linsley, 2000, p. 48). This chapter will describe the cycle of assaultive behavior and provide predictive factors for aggression and violence.

2. The assault cycle.

The assault cycle has distinct patterns that can assist in predicting violence and enable the health care professional to administer appropriate measures. The patterns in assaultive behavior are common in different groups, genders and persons. In every cycle, different behaviors can be observed in particular phases. The five phases of the assault cycle include: trigger, escalation, crisis, recovery phase and post crisis.

2.1.Trigger phase.

An individual begins to detect threats to their security or welfare. Feelings of being denied, being ignored or being refused something important to them crop in. The aggressor then becomes frustrated as Linsley (2006, p. 48) highlights.

A person in trigger phase perceives that they have lost control. They review the issues facing them and see the magnitude of the conflict as huge. Fear is real and the person in crisis endeavor to compensate what they are denied. They may be in denial and reason with self to justify events.

The trigger is as a result of other people's actions, an argument with another person, upsetting information an in- ability to do something they have been denied such as consuming alcohol or even a smoke break. Crisis can be eliminated if the problems and conflicts are solved. Trigger phase is not associated with experiences of medication or hallucinations.

Poor communication is experienced in the trigger phase. Interpersonal relations are poor and characterized by a great deal of tension. The person in crisis may try to control self from causing outburst and motivating another person to have an outburst.

The appropriate response towards the potentially aggressive person would be to divert their mind and destract them. Exercising good communication skills where one remains neutral would be helpful. A healthcare professional can alert others and record observations. The healthcare professional should remain calm and avoid showing signs of fear. Keep a distance, show the hands and stay close to exit.

2.2. Escalation phase.

The person in crisis begins to prepare for aggression. Threats are presented verbally to the prospective victim if they are within reach.

Anger steps in and the aggressor throws objects, begins pacing and kicking walls. The voice is raised and yelling that is sometime accompanied by banging is experienced or seen.

The escalating phase provides an opportunity for a healthcare professional trained in assaultive behavior to employ de- escalating techniques to prevent violence from occurring. If possible, explaining to the aggressive person that consequences of violence can be severe can be helpful. This can be done with caution because it can be perceived as a threat to the aggressor.

Adamowski et al (2009, p. 740) adds that, the thinking process is affected by the high levels of anger and distress. Consequently, the aggressor begins to become dysfunctional, disorganized and lacks sleep. They may direct their anger to animals or objects rather than directing them towards a person. Very minor events become a cause of argument.

When the healthcare professional recognizes escalating behavior, they should communicate to other professionals and ask for company. If the situation has the possibility of becoming violent they should notify the supervisor and avoid attending to the person alone. Showing fear, disappointment, impatience and annoyance may convey negative information to the aggressor. Hands should be kept where they can be seen and space between the aggressor and others should be maintained.

Negotiation and conversation with persons who are drunk and under influence of drugs should be avoided.

The security should be involved if the violent threat is imminent. Using communication skills for de-escalating violence to prevent the aggressor from becoming violent is necessary.

2.3.Crisis phase.

Crisis stage involves actual aggressive behavior. The aggressor assaults the seeming threat. A lot of energy is used in violence. The person in crisis becomes weary very quick because the energy to sustain an attack is limited.

In the crisis phase, the aggressor dominates the victim by controlling with violence. The abuser is unpredictable and fears losing power, therefore, they use violence to control. The aggressor believes it is the victim on the wrong. The victim of assaultive behavior is abused, feels helpless and becomes traumatized.

To ensure they have control, the abuser takes time to decide words to use and place they will use for abuse. They scheme and attempt to do what they have planned on the victim. Besides hurting the person they want to abuse, the assaultive person hurts pets and destroys property. In the mental health facility, they can throw chairs, over throw tables and physically attack staff or fellow patients.

The victim of violence blames self for suffering the violence because they might have contributed to causing violence. Alongside feeling terrified, the victim of abuse sense embarrassment, shame and humiliation. The victim experiences fear and shock. When attacked they should call for help.

This is an attempt to remove them from the trap (Chou et al, 2001, p. 139). The abuser refreshes the conflict and uses it as an excuse for punishing the victim. Punishing the victim gives the aggressor a short lived feeling that they have resolved the problem. The abuser becomes irrational and continues threats.

2.4.Recovery phase.
After becoming assaultive the aggressor slows down to recover. The aggressor is watchful and any impending threats could generate another assault. The feeling of being disorganized remains and the aggressor becomes confused. Some aggressors become depressed and commit crime against themselves such as self-injury and suicide.

In an attempt to recover what has been damaged, the aggressor reconciles by showing affection and apologizing. The abuser ends violence and demonstrates their desire to change. Because of feeling remorseful the aggressor becomes sad and shows that they are repentant.

In some cases the aggressor refuses to apologize and ignores the violent event. They leave the victim without saying a word and disappear. Some return and request the victim to sympathize with them. They become very convincing to justify their act and profess that they will not repeat assault. Ways of de-escalating violence can be implemented to prevent the aggressor from becoming violent again, and listen to the aggressor (Ford et al 2010, p. 74).

2.5.Post crisis phase.
The aggressive individual calms down and

becomes emotional about their actions. They show intense remorse, fatigue and despair. They begin to blame self and hide from others. The aggressor might begin crying, sleeping or just remain alone in a corner. The aggressor may attempt to mend their existing relationship with the victim. The post crisis is peaceful.

In some cases the aggressor does not have remorse and may be happy about the violence. What causes the cycle to begin is when interpersonal difficulties arise. When the interpersonal issues continue to add, the situation becomes different and tension begins to build; causing the cycle to start.

Positive talk and affirmation should be emphasized to decrease the chances of triggering another cycle of violence. The aggressor can engage in different activities like recreation and exercising to divert their mind. Mark the triggers of assault and avoid mentioning or accommodating them.

Reaching out for spiritual help and mediation from a skilled person can assist destabilize crisis (Salmon, 2007, p. 14).

3. Aggression and violent predictive factors.

As assaultive behavior continues to become a major concern in healthcare, researchers have engaged in discovering factors that can predict violence. The motive of conducting the research is to ensure the safety of the healthcare professionals as well as the patients and their families.

3.1. Demography and personal history.

In the healthcare facilities, demography and personal history play a major role in providing information on the possibility of aggressive behavior. Chapman et al (2009, p. 476) mention that, an individual who have shown threats of hostility and belong to a group or subculture that engages in violence could be a prospective violent person. Male patients are believed to have higher likelihood of becoming violent than women.

Healthcare professionals take into consideration the history of the patient, healthcare worker or visitor. Aggressive tendencies in the past can be identified as a possibility for aggression in the future. Incidents of cruelty towards self and others are used to determine the possibility of aggression. The presence of men as the majority in aggressive behavior may not be necessarily correct in relation to violent behavior in healthcare.

Young people tend to be involved in violence than older people. There is a correlation of low income earners, unemployed, low literacy levels being a contributive factor to violence.

Healthcare facilities report high cases of violence occur at night as opposed to the day. Aggressive people become violent towards the victim if the victim is alone and is female. When there is less surveillance from the hospital guards and visiting time for patients, violence tend to occur. When the aggressor sees that there is no security, they are likely to take the opportunity to exhibit violence. The frequency of assaultive behavior in a given population is used as a base line to predict violence. Use of rates of previous occurrence to predict is considered to be an actual factor.

3.2. Individual disorders, sickness and substance abuse factors.

The individual may be having personal crisis where they lost control or power. Anxiety disorder is regarded as a ground for causing aggression and can predict violence. The person causing violence may be using medication without a prescription. Delirium can cause violence if the patient has seizures, infection, and trauma or electrolyte imbalance (reversible). Brain injury, Dementia, excess alcohol and Alzheimer's disease can contribute to the development of aggressive behavior. Previous mental problems like paranoia, personality disorders, psychiatric illnesses or psychosis can predict violence.

When the person in crisis senses unmanageable powerlessness, humiliation and extreme fear, they may become violent as a way of controlling internal feelings. The desire is to defend them from danger and to gain control. Grieve is another factor that can cause an individual to become violent. A series of violence in the past can influence the person to become violent. Once they have become violent in the past, there is a tendency of becoming violent in the future.

Morrison et al (1998, p. 558) argue that attacks towards healthcare professional are not abrupt. Patients and healthcare professionals who become assaultive can be identified before they become violent. Prior to becoming violent, the aggressor will experience increasing tension, give threats and become stressed. History of violence is one of the reliable factors for predicting violence. Employment, literacy level, ethnicity and gender are weak factors for predicting violence.

Loss of trust for the physician, visitors, relatives and other healthcare professionals in the hospital can lead to wild suspicions that will inspire aggressive behavior. Provocation to cause violence is a situation that may eventually end up causing violence **(Belayachi et al, 2010, p. 27)**. Individuals who are unable to tolerate stress can become assaultive. People with psychiatric disorders such as schizophrenia, depression and bipolar together with schizoaffective disorder are prone to becoming aggressive.

Substance abuse and excessive consumption of alcohol is a prominent contributor of violence in healthcare facilities. Patients with mental disorders and the psychotic consuming alcohol have a higher tendency of becoming aggressive than those who do not consume alcohol or abuse substances.

3.3. Situational factors.

Ferns (2006, p. 42) states that, situations that facilitate occurrence of violence can be used as a predictive factor. The availability of weapons such as knives, guns, sharp objects where the person in crisis can access them could lead to aggressive behavior. The presence of a person who stimulates the feeling of injustice, oppression as well as inequality can trigger abuse. When the person is forced to feel threatened and defenseless they become aggressive. Individuals who have experienced abuse from self or others in the past can quickly become aggressive if same condition is applied to the present.

If the person feels isolated from the rest of the people and is removed from their place of comfort without consent, they may not welcome the change and instead become aggressive. When something unexpected occurs, the event can stimulate anger which can eventually erupt into violence. There are prevailing circumstances that encourage violence such as overcrowding, favors towards others and uninformed rules.

Healthcare facilities have been used as a holding place for detainees and people serving a jail term when the correctional institutions are crowded. People who are brought to hospital are mentally disturbed, sick and aggressive. The emergency rooms have people who are under the influence of drugs. The police let the people stay in the emergency rooms until they become sober. When in the hospital the detainees, people under influence of drugs and the ill can become aggressive to self, other patients, healthcare providers and other people within reach.

Antisocial personalities predispose to violence. The person disregards others and does not pay attention to other people's rights. The antisocial personalities who are mentally ill are likely to relapse and engage in substance use. Psychopathic personality is another predictive factor where the aggressor is self-centered and brutal.

3.4. Actuarial and clinical predictive factors.

Prediction of aggressive behavior or violence has been given different approaches to include clinical actuarial and structured methods. Predicting violence has been seen as a very challenging task because assaultive behavior has occurred even in circumstances where no risk had been detected. Actuarial methods of predicting violence take into considerations risk factors such as diagnosis, psychopathological condition, gender and age (statistical assessment). Actuarial methods predicted violence if the same patient is exposed to same conditions in the future. As a result, the method does not recognizing the judgment of the healthcare professional dealing with the current situation and is often used for admitted patients. Data collected on the specific patient is used to make the judgment if the person is likely to become aggressive. Clinical methods of predicting violence have been used to predict overt behavior and consider factors such as psychopathology. Clinical methods are structured and assessment is done according to situation.

3.5. Broset violence registers.

Abderhalden et al (2006, p. 17) state that prediction of assaultive behavior is possible during routine care. Healthcare professionals can forecast violence using the violence register on a short term basis.

Violence check list consist of six observations of the possible aggressive person. The observations include irritation, confusion, abusive and threatening words, and boisterousness, attacking animals and objects and physical threats. When the six observations are recorded, there is a higher probability of the person to become violent.

4. Conclusion.

The assault cycle begins with a trigger when behavior of a person changes and tension begins to build up. The next cycle is escalation phase where the body and verbal words reveal unmanageable anger. The next phase is crisis where the aggressive person acts violently. After the crisis the aggressor enters recovery phase when they begin calming down. The final phase is post crisis phase where the assaultive person becomes remorseful. In an attempt to resolve issues the aggressor and victim can disagree leading to a trigger; hence the cycle begins again. This must be avoided. Ways of de-escalating violence should be exercised to prevent assaultive behavior. Aggression and violent predictive factors include: Demographic (age, gender), history, disorders, sickness and use of substance, situational (prevailing circumstances), Actuarial, clinical, and Broset violence register predictive factors.

References

Abderhalden, C. A., Needham, I., Dassen, T., Halfens, R., Haug, H. J., and Fischer, J. (2006)   Predicting inpatient violence using an extended version of the Brøset-Violence-Checklist: instrument development and clinical application. *Bio Med Central Psychiatry*, 6, 17.

Adamowski, T., Piotrowski, P., Trizna, M., and Kiejna, A. (2009). Assessment of types and incidence of aggression among patients admitted due to aggressive behaviors, *Psychiatry Pol* 43(6), 739- 749.

Belayachi, J., Berrechid, K., Amlaiky, F., Zekraoui, A., and **Abouqa**, R. (2010). Violence toward physicians in emergency departments of Morocco: prevalence, predictive factors, and psychological impact. JOURNAL OF OCCUPATIONAL MEDICINE AND TOXICOLOGY **5**, 27.

Chapman, R. Perry, L., Styles, I., and Combs, S. (2009). Predicting patient aggression against   nurses in all hospital areas, British journal of Nursing, 18(8), 476-483.

Chou, K. R., Lu, R. B., and Chang, M. (2001). Assaultive behavior by psychiatric in-patient and its related factors. *Journal of Nursing Research,* 9 (15), 139- 151.

Ferns, T. (2006) Violence, aggression and physical assault in healthcare settings. *Nursing   Standard,* 13, 42.

Ford, K., Byrt, R and James, D. (2010). Preventing and Reducing Aggression and Violence in   Health and Social Care: A Holistic Approach. UK: M&K Update Ltd

Linsley, P. (2006). *Violence and Aggression in the Workplace: A Practical Guide for All   Healthcare Staff.* Abingdon: Radcliffe Publishing.

Morrison, J. L., Lantos, J. D., Levinson, W. (1998). Aggression and Violence Directed Toward
     Physicians. *Journal of general Internal medicine,* 13(8), 556- 561.

Salmon, N., and Varela, R. (2007) *Learning to manage assaultive behavior.* New York: AMN   Healthcare Services Inc.

Crisis Intervention and Prevention in Healthcare
Questions Chapter 3

1. The patterns in assaultive behavior are common in different groups, genders and persons

   True
   False

2. Which of the following include the five phases of the assault cycle

   A. Post crisis

   B. Trigger

   C. Crisis

   D. All of the above

3. Conflict can be eliminated if the problems and conflicts are solved

   True
   False

4. Good communication is experience in the trigger phase

   True
   False

5. In the escalating phase anger steps in and the aggressor throws objects, begins pacing and kicks walls

   True

False

6. In this phase anger may be directed to animals or objects rather than directing them to a person

   A. Trigger

   B. Escalating

   C. Crisis

   D. Recovery

7. Negotiation and conversation with persons who are drunk and under influence of drugs should be avoided

   True
   False

8. In which of the following phase the aggressor dominates the victim by controlling with violence

   A. Trigger

   B. Escalating

   C. Recovery

   D. Crisis

9. The aggressor is watchful and any impending threats could generate another assault in the _____ phase

   A. Trigger

B. Escalating

C. Recovery

D. Crisis

10. in which of the following phase the aggressor might begin crying sleeping or just remain alone in a corner

A. Post crisis

B. Crisis

C. Trigger

D. Escalating

11. Assaultive behavior is no longer a major concern in healthcare

True
False

12. In the healthcare facilities demography and personal history play a major role in providing information on the possibility of aggressive behavior

True
False

13. Male patients are believed to have lower likelihood of becoming violent than women

True
False

14. Young people tend to be involved in violence than older people

True

False

15. Healthcare facilities report high cases of violence occur at night as opposed to the day

True

False

16. Violence tend to occur when there is less surveillance from the hospital guards and visiting time for patients

True

False

17. _____ can cause violence if the patient has seizures, infection and trauma or electrolyte imbalance

A. Anxiety

B. Delirium

C. Dementia

D. Alzheimer's

18. Employment, literacy level, ethnicity and gender are major factors for predicting violence

True

False

19. When a person is force to feel threatened and defenseless they become aggressive

True

False

20. Antisocial personalities which are personal traits can predict violence

True
False

Chapter Four

1. Introduction.

2. Obtaining patient history from a patient with violent behaviors

2.1.Identifying sources of information

2.2.Preparing

2.3.Eliminate triggers of aggressive behavior and use appropriate communication skills

2.4.Gathering the information

2.5.Identify common issues.

3. Characteristics of aggressive and violent patients and victims

3.1.Emotional and behavioral characteristics

3.2.Physical characteristics

3.3.Personality characteristics

3.4.Relationship with others

3.5.Medical and substance use analysis

4. Conclusion

Crisis prevention and Intervention in healthcare
1. Introduction.

Healthcare professionals require the information of a patient with assaultive behavior to prevent and intervene in the event of crisis. This information is used in the implementation of appropriate preventive measures. Additionally, the traits of patients and victims of assaultive behavior should be recognized to assist the patient and the victim accordingly. This chapter will discuss how patient history with violent behaviors is obtained. It will also provide the characteristic of aggressive and violent patients and victims.

2. Obtaining patient history from a patient with violent behaviors.

The history of an aggressive and violent patient can be difficult to obtain if there is no record. Hospital records can be handy when gathering information. The patient history enable the healthcare professionals give the most accurate intervention in a given situation. Obtaining a patients history can be viewed as a process that facilitates accumulation of information.

2.1.Identifying sources of information.

Obtaining information from patients with aggressive behaviors may be challenging because the aggressive patients are not usually willing to cooperate and disseminate negative information about themselves. *By the way, who will like to say something bad about themselves?*

77

The information can be obtained from family members, medical records, friends, and the police as well as healthcare workers. Some patients may be willing to provide information and be involved in the decision making and should be allowed. Family members may be a good source of information on how current events happened and how past events occurred. Friends of the violent patient can give additional information on behavior, for example, if they have been substance abusers. Some of the friends, family members, members of the public may have been victims of assaultive behavior caused by the individual. The police may have current and past history about criminal activities and arrests. The medical record is a reliable source of information (Dubin, 1993, p. 10).

McNeil et al (2011, p. 23) submits that, the healthcare professionals should record all the information concerning the patient and then keep the record. If there are no existing medical records in the healthcare facility the healthcare professional may have to get information from family, friends or the public. Observing and questioning the patient could help generate information.

2.2.Preparing.

The history of a patient behavior and condition is very significant when it comes to making decisions on healthcare practice and should be conducted when the healthcare professional is ready.

Eichelman and Hartwig (1995, p. 84) suggest that, before attempting to gain the information from the violent patient, prepare self by clearing what is in the mind. If the records are available, the health care provider can view the last significant problem presented. Consider the available time for obtaining the information and if it is the correct timing.

Develop a strategy to use in case the patient becomes violent. Handle the circumstances with confidence and calmness. Information should be sought after the patient and the healthcare professional are calm. Get ready for responses void of argument and heated disputes. The healthcare professional can acknowledge the upsetting situation the patient is experiencing and assure them of assisting them. Plan to distract the attention of aggressive patient. Eliminate situations where the patient might feel confronted.

Prepare self by ensuring that you are in good health and ready before beginning obtaining information from the patient. The healthcare professional should deal with emotions that emanate from past experiences when dealing with an assaultive patient.

Past experiences can cause distress and scare the healthcare professional. Obtain support and manage the experiences immediately after the incident and find a long term solution. Discuss with other professionals to prevent anger and temperament. Depending on the circumstances, the healthcare professional can ask another worker for company. Moreover, choose an appropriate environment.

2.3.Eliminate triggers of aggressive behavior and use appropriate communication skills.

From observation made when the patient is aggressive, identify events that led to aggressiveness. These could include frustration, intrusion to the patient's privacy, anxiety, fear, feeling threatened, discomfort, and pain. Manage their pain and avoid abrupt movement or noise. Avoid all the triggers that could lead to assault. They can be made comfortable by giving appropriate meals and adequate drinks. Keep away from rushing them to do something and giving demands. Explain actions before you attend to them, give simple explanation and give them time to give an answer. Do not show when offended and evade criticizing the patient.

Gathering information requires the healthcare professional to use appropriate communication skills. Both verbal and non verbal skills matter. The physical distance between the patient and healthcare professional should be safe. Stay confident and calm when gathering information from the violent patient. An apology for waiting for long at the beginning is appreciated. Address the patient properly while showing respect. The healthcare professional can listen to the patient and avoid writing or getting distracted when what the aggressive/violent patient is saying something of relevance to them. If there is need to write, notify them and allow them to complete talking. Take note of topics and activities that interest the patient and use them when necessary to call for their attention. Be a good listener and ask all relevant information without offending the patient.

2.4.Gathering the information.

Obtaining data from patients may take different forms when the healthcare professional begins obtaining information. They may give single-word answers, may present themselves with a self-diagnosis and demand for medication, may need continuous reassurance, and may be angry or show tendencies of assaultive behavior.

Questions can be effective in gathering information if they are not leading. Polite steering of phrases can also help get information. Reassure the patient of confidentiality at all times. Avoid interrupting the patient when giving their first statement (Kanel 2012, p. 33). An example is a patient that came into a mental health facility claiming that he was God. His delusion of grandiose was so strong that he was narrating his experience when he was being crucified, told us how he was so exhausted before Joseph of Aramathea came to help him carry the cross to Calvary. As we obtained data during his admission, one of the questions was "Do you have problem with anger?". He was asked the question and immediately he bursted out into a very loud and infectious laughter, laughing so hard and finally ended up asking us, the nurses "Does God have problem with anger?". We could not control ourselves in a hearty laughter! But after the laughter, we continued to obtain the needed information.

Information sought consists of demographics, which includes their age, gender and marital status. Find out if they have social support from friends, family or community.

Get details of their involvement in previous assaults, abuse of substance or alcohol and other sicknesses. Check and record physical traits that may imply involvement in aggressive behavior or crisis. Additionally, record verbal indicators that suggest the patient is in crisis.

The healthcare professional should remain focused when questioning the patient, relatives, friend, other healthcare professionals, and police as well as when looking for relevant material. Concentrating and focusing on causes, concerns, and underlying issues that necessitated the patient's visit to the hospital is essential. Focusing will cause the healthcare professional to make appropriate observation. The patient and their family or friends at times need reassurance and confirmation, which should be received well. Patient-tailored assessment gives the healthcare professionals ability to identify the needs of the patient and their anticipation.

According to Tardiff (1996, p. 141), a patient has a right to give consent since they are responsible for their well-being. The healthcare professional has a duty to examine, treat and eliminate risks that are related to medicine. The patient has to consent so that the healthcare professional is capable of assisting the patient. The patient is required to provide the healthcare professional with compelling information about their condition.

2.5. Identify common issues.

After conducting the search on the patient with aggressive and violent behavior, a record of the observations and information obtained should be documented.

This will be useful in the future, especially in the coordination of patient care. Information obtained will reveal what causes or triggers the violence, intervention that is given and the effectiveness.

The information makes it possible to identify underlying issues that need to be addressed. Issues that are unique to the patient are identified. The information will give details of social history, medical history, family history, use of drugs and excessive use of alcohol.

3. **Characteristics of aggressive and violent patients and victims.**

3.1.Emotional and behavioral characteristics.

Shepherd (2001, p. 114) states that aggressive patients may show negative emotions such as anger, discontentment and anxiety. The patient is very irritable and unfriendly. The assaultive patient could be frustrated from present, ongoing and future events they have no control over. The violent patients show signs of withdrawal if they have been abusing substance or alcohol.

Common behaviors that violent people have include constant desire to call for attention. Violent patients show traits such as agitation and restlessness. A violent patient has fear and emotional attachment in their conversation. Assaultive patients have an augmented motor activity. Violent patients are often disorderly, antisocial and disruptive.

Consequently, aggressive patients may become confused and become wild. The victim of emotional and behavioral assaults may feel devalued or dehumanized. Poor communication will cause hostility and misunderstanding.

3.2.Physical characteristics.

The violent patient uses verbal or physical abuse towards self, healthcare professionals, relatives, non-relatives, animals or objects. Patients with assaultive behavior could be young adults in their early twenties or teenagers. Although majority of violent patients are young, there are elderly patients who become violent. Both men and women could possess assaultive behavior traits. Although it is worth noting that majority are men, Women cannot be underestimated especially in the case of mental illnesses. Patients with violence might have had head injury and trauma. A violent patient may have a weapon, or objects that can inflict pain on others. Both fresh and old wounds may be seen on the violent person skin.

Aggressive patients use inappropriate physical contact to inflict harm on self and others. They use force to slap, bit, bite, spit and kick. The physical actions of a patient with assaultive behavior includes using unacceptable contact to create a situation that is uncomfortable and hostile. Victims of physical assault fear the aggressor. While some may have tendencies of revenge, others will leave the aggressive patient to be attended by others. The victim may have sustained injuries and need medical care.

3.3.Personality characteristics.

Aggressive patients have a low level of tolerance when they are frustrated. Violent patients at times reject criticism and want to be in control. They tend to blame others for faulty results that involve others or self. Patients with violent personality may engage in antisocial behavior, selfishness, careless driving and egocentricity.

Patients with low intellectual abilities can become violent when compared with the intelligent patients. Patients from low social and economic status tend become assaultive when compared with those from a high social status. Assaultive patients are characterized by brutal behavior, intimidating actions and words together with yelling to scold others. Violent patients have a poor judgment (Tardiff, 1996, p. 27). Violent patients may be comfortable with the assaultive behavior and live it as a lifestyle. In this case, the aggressive patient does not have remorse. Insults and aggressive behavior is used as a way of manipulating others.

As a result, the aggressive person becomes involved in breaking laws. Some patients with violence had been trained on violence as police or military officers.

3.4.Relationship with others.

Aggressive patients tend to have poor relationships with the healthcare professional as well as the other patients. The assaultive patient may try to convince and take the other to an activity. The communication is very poor and they do not communicate effectively. Other patients who are calm tend to dissociate themselves from them.

The aggressive patient may want to intrude the personal or physical space of the healthcare professional, other patients, relatives or friends disturbing the existing peace. The patient may react negatively towards treatment, relatives or assistance. They may retaliate if they feel not treated right. Violent patients may perceive others as being in competition and fail to cooperate when granted help. The aggressive patient can provoke and tease unspecific patients, relatives, friends or healthcare professionals in the healthcare facility.

The healthcare professionals need to re-emphasize the rules of the unit and state the consequences of breaking those rules. It is paramount to remind the residents of the mental health unit that the staff are their friends and are working in the facility to ensure the improvement of their health status. Since the presence of a poor relationship between the staff and the patient makes the potentially assaultive patient to become violent, the healthcare professional needs to ensure that adequate communication exists between the two parties and proper and therapeutic techniques are being utilized to ensure a very conducive environment.

3.5.Medical and substance use traits

Tardiff (1999, p. 153) mentions that, mentally ill patients are likely to become violent. Patient with bipolar disorder, depression and schizophrenia tend to engage in violence. Similarly, patients who abuse substance and alcohol are at times violent. Paranoid patients and those with hallucinations can become violent.

Violent patients may have depression, accompanied with hopelessness and suicidal tendencies. This occurs if treatment has not exerted remarkable improvement or if the patient does not adhere to the medication regimen.

The victim of violence becomes fearful and anxious after they experience assault. Their confidence and self-esteem is affected which could lead to a withdrawal from giving support or adequate healthcare to the patient. The victim of violence attempts to change behavior and please the aggressive patient to avoid being victimized again. The victims tend to withdraw and blame self for the aggressor's violence. The victim becomes tensed and guilty. They are terrified and may want to run away. In some cases, they may want to defend self by inflicting harm on the patient. Other victims feel ashamed because they were helpless and not able to change situation. Healthcare professionals who have experienced violence may not want to continue working with the identified violent patients. If persuaded to work, they may demand that the patient is strictly cautioned about causing violence and verbal abuse. Injuries or bruises from the assault may cause indignity on the victim. Victims who are counseled anticipate that the patient will change (Blumenreich and Lewis, 1993, 22).

Healthcare professional victims who have encountered violent patients are pre-disposed to making medical errors and failing to satisfy patients' healthcare needs. Scared victims excuse themselves from working. The motivation to work for the same unit is negatively affected especially if the violent patient is not responding to treatment.

87

Victims of assault become stressed over personal safety. Stress can cause the victim to begin abusing drugs and consuming alcohol. Healthcare professionals caring for violent patients tend to ask for some leave from work. Burnout has been diagnosed on healthcare professionals, friends and family members of the aggressive patients. They may have stereotypes and believe in social myths about image. The victim's self-image is low. They shun away from interacting with others and want to remain isolated. Because of trauma and fear, victims of violence may lack sleep (Kemshall and Pritchard, 2000, p. 109).

Victims of assaultive behavior may become defensive for any critic from abuser. They lose interest in the existing relationship with the abuser. In extreme cases victims of violence may attempt to commit suicide or harm self. Victims of assaultive behavior need special attention and counselling. They require support and help. One should consider the relationship of the aggressor and victim before taking legal action against the aggressor. Violent patients have caused disability, permanent injuries and even death to the victims (Graham 1998, p. 135).

4. Conclusion.

History of patients with aggressive and violent behavior can be obtained by identifying sources of information. Information can be obtained from the patient, relatives, friends, police, observation and medical records. Once the source is identified the healthcare professional can prepare self psychologically and physically.

Get rid of triggers of aggressive behavior and apply appropriate communication skills. Gather the information by focusing on relevant information and get the patient's consent. Identify common issues and keep and record. Violent patients are characterized by negative emotions and behavior. They may be physically aggressive and have personality traits of exhibiting violence. They have poor relationships with other people, may have mental illness or use drugs. Victims of violence have fear, anger, blame self, are terrified and make effort to run away. Victims may have depression, low self-esteem and negative self-image. Some have injuries and tendencies of revenge. If not assisted, victims may hurt self or die from injuries.

References
Blumenreich, P. and Lewis, S. (1993). *Management of the Violent Patient in the Treatment   Setting.* New York: Routledge.

Dubin, W. R. (1993). *Clinician Safety.* American Psychiatric Association. Task Force on   Clinician Safety.

Eichelman, B. S. and Hartwig, A. C. (1995). *Patient Violence & the Clinician.* Washington, DC:
     American Psychiatric Press.

Graham, A., Hamberger, L. K., and Burge, S. K. (1998). *Violence Issues for Health Care   Educators and Providers.* Binghamton, NY:The Haworth Press.

Kanel, K. (2012). *A Guide to Crisis Intervention.* Belmont, CA: Congen Learning.

Kemshall, H. and Pritchard, J. (2000). *Good Practice in Working with Victims of Violence.*   Philadelphia, PA: Jessica Kingsley.

McNeil, D. E., Hung, E. K., Cramer, R. J., Hall, S. E., Binder, R. L. (2011).An approach to   Evaluating Competence in Assessing and Managing Violent Risk. *Psychiatric Services,*   62(1)

Shepherd, J. (2001). *Violence in Health Care: Understanding, Preventing and Surviving   Violence: A Practical Guide for Health Professionals.* Oxford: OUP Oxford.

Tardiff, K. (1996).*Concise Guide to Assessment and Management of Violent Patients, Second   Edition.* Washington, DC: American Psychiatric Press.

Tardiff, K. (1999). *Medical Management of the Violent Patient: Clinical Assessment and   Therapy.* New York: Marcel Dekker.

Crisis Intervention and Prevention in Healthcare
Questions Chapter 4

1. Family members may be a good source of information on how current events happened and how past events occurred

   True
   False

2. The medical record is not a reliable source of information

   True
   False

3. Eichelman and Hartwig suggest that before attempting to gain information from a violent patient prepare self by clearing what is in the mind

   True
   False

4. Only verbal skills matter when eliminating triggers of aggressive behavior

   True
   False

5. A patient has a right to give consent since they are responsible for their well-being

   True
   False

6. The history of an aggressive and violent patient can be easy to obtain if there is no records

True
False

7. Information obtained will reveal what causes or triggers the violence, intervention that is given and the effectiveness

True
False

8. Violent patients show traits such as agitation and restlessness

True
False

9. Victim of emotional and behavioral assaults may feel devalued or dehumanized

True
False

10. The majority of violent patients are young adults in their early twenties

True
False

11. Aggressive patients have a high level of tolerance when they are frustrated

True
False

12. Patients with low intellectual abilities can become violent when compared with the intelligent patients

True
False

13. Insults and aggressive behavior is used as a way of manipulating others

True
False

14. Aggressive patient tend to have poor relationships with the healthcare professional as well as the other patients

True
False

15. Violent patients may perceive others as being in competition and fail to cooperate when granted help

True
False

16. Assaultive patients are characterized by brutal behavior

True
False

17. Patient with bipolar disorder, depression and schizophrenia tend to engage in violence

True
False

18. Victims of assaultive behavior do not get stressed over personal safety

True
False

19. According to Kemshall and Pritchard substance abuse victims may lack sleep because of trauma and fear

True
False

20. Victims of assaultive behavior need special attention and counseling

True
False

Chapter Five

Outline

Introduction
1. Verbal and physical maneuvers to diffuse and avoid

    violent behavior

1.1 Non-verbal and verbal communication

1.2 Tension de-escalation

1.3 Anger de-escalation

1.4 Substance abuse de-escalation

1.5 Physical maneuvers

2. Strategies to avoid physical harm

3.1.Escape from behind chocking

3.2.Stance and Front chocking

3.3.Release of arms

3.4.Punching, biting and pulling the hair

3.5.Patients with weapons

Conclusion

Crisis prevention and Intervention in healthcare

1. Introduction.

Crisis in healthcare is unfavorable and could compromise the outcomes of medical intervention as well as create new challenges. Putting off the chances of a crisis occuring could be life threatening. There is need to protect self from injuries that can cause decline in motivation and physical injury resulting from aggressive behavior. To expose valuable ways of handling crisis, this chapter discusses physical maneuvers to diffuse and avoid violent behavior. It also explains strategies that can be used to avoid physical harm.

2. Verbal and physical maneuvers to diffuse and avoid violent behavior.

In managing assaultive behavior different ways of diffusing and de-escalating assaultive behavior are applied in an effort to prevent violence. De-escalating assaultive behaviors require the use of techniques when an incident is likely to occur to prevent assaults.

2.1.Non -verbal and verbal communication.

Clear and effective communication when dealing with the patient with assaultive behavior should be adopted. When responding to patients, communicate verbally and write down the instructions that support conversation to rule out chances of misunderstanding.

Clear explanation at the beginning of the therapeutic relationship or when conducting a procedure helps the patient to know what to expect while helping the nurse obtain what they need. (Glick et al, 2008 p. 126).

Leather (1999, p. 169) reveals that to create and communicate boundaries about treatment and contact is an effective way of diffusing assaultive behavior. Explain what to expect and outcomes of staying in hospital, whether staying for long or for a short time. If a patient has been placed on a 72-hour hold, 14-day hold, 30-day hold, etc., the patient should have a clear idea as to how long they are staying and the reason for the mental health evaluation hold. Be consistent in recording decisions and incidents in the hospital. If the client is to be transferred to another facility, proper communication is necessary, as well.

When talking to the patient ask questions that are open ended and give adequate time to the patient to think and give a response. Respect the patient's space. When the assaultive patients asks questions, explain in very simple but direct language. Avoid giving answers you are not sure. Use very simple words and short sentences when talking or responding.

While the patient is conversing, allow them to vent their opinions. Direct eye contact, nodding of head, etc assures the patient that you are still interested in the conversation. Be neutral and avoid smiling unnecessarily which can be easily mistaken for mockery and stimulate anxiety. Keep away from touching the patient while talking.

Reaching out while talking to the aggressive person can be translated as a threat, even though it could be a habit that one is accustomed to when talking (Forester, 1997, p.42).

When they are yelling and talking in loud voice, do not scream to be heard. Remain calm until they take a breath, then talk to the aggressive person calmly. Be selective in responding to questions and attempt to answer the questions. Questions asked can be rudely presented; however, the healthcare professional should be willing to answer. Abusive questions should be ignored and not answered. Explain rules politely. Empathy is shown and not inappropriate behavior. The healthcare professional should practice self-control to avoid giving threats and showing that they are angry.

2.2. Tension de-escalation.

In managing assaultive behavior the voice used should be polite, low tone and confident. Avoid talking when the patient is irritable. In their study, Holmes et al (2013, p. 271) found out that the healthcare professional can manage behavior and avoid being inflexible. The body language can be controlled to avoid stimulating anxiety. A safe distance can be kept between the healthcare professional and the aggressive patient. Address the patient using their name and use own name.

It is wise to obtain the patient's consent before administering medication or giving medical examination. Use clear words and attempt to clearly understand their response.

Pay attention and listen carefully to every response they give. Be specific when asking and requesting for targeted answers. When conversing, avoid making promises. The healthcare professionals can express their desire to help. Assist the patient in expressing their thoughts and divert them from issues causing tension.

The situation should be assessed and de-escalating techniques employed before the patient progresses to becoming assaultive. Tension de-escalation can be achieved by attempting to solve the problem at the moment. The healthcare professional can show empathy and give help if requested. Tension can be reduced by assuring the patient that they are not in danger and will not be hurt. Engaging the patient in a conversation or activity to divert their mind could help. Breathing exercises and relaxation can reduce tension.

2.3. Anger de-escalation.

Duxbury and Whittington (2004, p. 476) mention that when anger is not managed it can soar into violence. When the patient's anger is constantly increasing it may be necessary to walk away and give the patient time to calm down. Let the patient vent and do not interrupt when they are angry. Be sincere when asked questions. After obtaining opportunities to have conversations assure them of confidentiality and seek for their agreement.

In some cases it is wise to agree to differ in opinion. Refuse to give in to defensive positions and encourage the patient to cooperate with the assistance being offered. Healthcare professionals can keep quiet or walk away if there are chances of engaging in an argument. Help the patient identify the underlying issues that are causing them to be angry. Healthcare professionals can facilitate boundaries that are practical and participate in implementing them. Avoid a situation that makes the patient sense interrogation.

Be firm on the boundaries set and show respect. If verbally assaulted remain calm and shun away from being defensive. Call for back up if caught up in a crisis. One can call for help or leave if de-escalation is not working. Hands should be visible so that it is easy to use them when needed. Putting hands in the pocket may be viewed as an attempt to take a weapon. Use hands appropriately without pointing or shaking fingers.

2.4.Substance abuse de-escalation.

Patients who show assaultive behavior and are under the influence of substance can be challenging to handle. Handling them requires patience. The patient can be given time to calm.
Examine the area and space and ensure they are safe for the patient and the healthcare professional. When they engage in a conversation, seek to understand them and let them know what others feel. Keep away from the patients who have abused drugs and reduce the frequency of dealing with them. Remain proactive and be positive when it comes to assisting them. It may be impossible to agree, still arguments should not be accommodated.

2.5.Physical maneuvers.

The healthcare professionals can acquire knowledge on how to deal with the assaultive behavior incidents in their area of specialization. Functional alarms can be installed at accessible positions in the hospital. The furniture can be designed such that there are no sharp ends and they cannot be used as a weapon. The layout of the hospital should be designed in a way that does not allow congestion and overcrowding of patients, visitors and healthcare professionals in a limited space. The rooms, corridors and facilities in the hospital should be ventilated and have enough lighting.

Additionally, avoid showing your back to the patient at any time. The healthcare professional should ensure they are placed between the patient and the exit. The way to the exit should be clear from obstruction. The eye level of the patients and the healthcare professional should be at equivalent level. The healthcare professional should stand if the patient is standing and request the patients to sit down so that they sit down. There should be space between patient and the healthcare professional such that the patient cannot stretch their arm and touch the other person. The healthcare professional should not be directly in front of the patient but at an angle. This will enable the healthcare professional to escape in case of an attack.

3. Strategies to avoid physical harm.

When developing strategies against physical harm take note of predictive factors and stay alert to take action when exposed to assaultive behavior.

101

When attempts to communicate and de-escalate assaultive behavior are ineffective, STOP! Safety is a priority and help should be sought after by leaving, calling for back up and informing your supervisor. Physical means are used as the final remedy. Strategies to avoid physical harm entail finding practical ways to escape or protecting body from injury.

3.1.Escape from behind chocking.

When attacked from behind gather confidence and remain calm and attempt to be in control. Raise both hands above the head. Then, twist to make the attacker lose their grip. While the hands are raised, twist towards the direction of the exit.

The legs should be twisted too to ease mobility. The healthcare professional that is attacked can twist hands downwards towards the completion of the twist to make the attacker arms unstable. Upon release, move quickly towards the exit, and call the security for assistance right away. Release self by turning if the attacker has chocked from behind and ensure the hands are lifted to make the attacker loose balance and grip.

3.2.Stance and Front chocking.

According to Bowie (2009, p. 64), it is appropriate to keep the legs apart and wide, as well as leave the arms open when standing. There should be distance between the patient and healthcare professional. When the attacker is aiming at the head, keep hands crossed over the head for protection. Deflect towards the flow when the aggressor gives a blow.

An aggressor who is kicking can be difficult to handle. The victim can protect self by turning body so that the kick hits the lateral area of the feet.

If the aggressor has attacked from the front, avoid backing up and continue being calm. Raise the hands higher than the head, a move which can confuse the attacker. A space between the shoulder and the neck is created when the hands are raised, causing the attacker to struggle with keeping the grip firm. Begin turning the feet towards the direction of the exit and then the body. While twisting the shoulders turn the hands downwards against the aggressor's hands; this will make the aggressive patient let go.

Protect the head from being hit when attacked, by covering with arms, boards or pillow (Bowie 2009, p. 64). Use the legs and feet to push away and prevent the aggressive patient from further attacking if one has fallen down. The arms of the healthcare professional can be twisted towards the attacker if their arms have been gripped by the aggressor. The face and throat should be protected at all times from being attacked. It is wise to master ways of avoiding the blows from reaching eyes and nose.

3.3.Release of arms.

The patient can hold the healthcare professional arms tightly and refuse to let go. It is normal to pull or try to drag away, but this will not help. The most appropriate way to cause an aggressor to let go of the arm is by pushing the hand downward rapidly closest to the floor. Once the aggressor's grip of the hand becomes weak, quickly rush towards the escape route.

After being free, keep off and call for help (Shepherd, 2001, p. 117).

The healthcare workers can use certain facility accepted codes to define the kind of attack and when they need assistance. In case the patient is stronger than the victim, the victim can plead for mercy. Asking for mercy and crying can contribute to release, and can be used instead of yelling or becoming aggressive towards the attacker. But this is the last resort.

3.4.Punching, biting and pulling the hair.
When the aggressor is punching, protect self by preventing them with an elevated shoulder together with the elbow.
Moreover, the elbow along with wrist can also be used to block punches. As the aggressor punches move towards their fist to destabilize them. Duxbury (2000, p. 111) suggests that when the aggressor bites, avoid pulling. Bites can be eliminated safely by pushing inside the mouth for them to release. When the aggressor bites push the bite towards the aggressors head in addition to holding their head. When the hair is pulled, make an effort to get hold of the aggressor's hands and direct them towards the head. Change direction by bending to the front to make them lose balance. If the hair is pooled from the front, contain hair by pulling closer to the scalp and then twist to the front facing downwards. Hair that is pulled can be released by holding the aggressors hands and pushing them down.

3.5.Patients with weapons.

Some patients may be armed with guns, knives and objects that can cause injury. To avoid physical harm it necessary to stay away from them. If staying away is impossible. the healthcare professional should not reach out for the weapon. Being careful is emphasized. Stay clear of fighting back.

If the attacker has a sharp object and attempts to stab or hit, hold their wrists. Hold the weapon with the right hand and use the left hand to gauge their eyes. This exercise requires agility. Move to the attackers back and pull their jaw to the left while attempting to make the aggressor lie down. Let the head of the aggressor go between the healthcare professional's knees. They can twist thumb and arm to take control of the weapon. If the aggressor is holding a weapon discuss with them and keep distance. Eyes should be kept on the aggressor. When the aggressive patient is holding a gun at a distance, escape by running in wavy or zigzag line and duck if possible. Shouting and yelling to the attacker might not help. Avoid struggling to fight and try to prevent the aggressor from causing injury to the victim or the aggressor.

Fauteux (2011, p. 199) insists that, healthcare professionals who are attacked by patients, workers or visitors can use self-defense techniques to protect the body from harm. They can shout for help and run away from violent person as quickly as possible. Healthcare professionals can consider taking self-defense classes to acquire the skill. Collaborating with other co-workers to work together and defend one another is important.

105

Following an attack, it is important to report to relevant authorities. Wykes (1994, p. 51), states that reporting is necessary because others could be in danger of being attacked. Moreover, the patient may need medical attention. The healthcare professional can report to immediate supervisor and should be examined. They may need attention because of being emotionally affected and require treatment if they were injured. The healthcare professional can be released to rest if they have been affected by the incident or sustained injuries.

4. Conclusion.

Diffusing violent behaviors involves using appropriate verbal and non-verbal language when communicating with a potentially violent person. It also involves listening, creating boundaries, and showing empathy. Violence can be diffused using techniques such as tension de-escalation, anger de-escalation and substance abuse de-escalation. De-escalation of violence is achieved by using correct tone and volume when speaking, avoiding confrontation, walking away, calling for help and letting the patient vent. Healthcare professionals show respect and remain patient when diffusing violence.

Physical maneuvers to diffuse and avoid violence entail installing alarms at accessible points, good lighting, avoid overcrowding and use furniture that cannot be exploited as a weapon in the healthcare facility. Keep distance and stay close to exit.

Strategies to avoid physical harm involve escaping and avoiding the aggressive person. One can free self if they are being chocked, held on the arm, bitten, punched or hair is pulled. One should avoid showing their back and standing close to the aggressive person.

References

Bowie, V (2009). Coping with violence: A guide for the human services. USA: Whiting and Burch Ltd.

Duxbury, J. and Whittington, R. (2004). Causes and management of patient aggression and violence: staff and patient perspectives. *Journal of Advanced Nursing,* 50(5), 469- 478.

Duxbury, J. (2000). *Difficult Patients.* Oxford: Reed Educational and Professional Publishing Ltd.

Fauteux, K. (2011). Defusing Angry People: Practical Tools for Handling Bullying, Threats, and Violence. New Jersey: New Horizon Press.

Forester, S. (1997). *The A-Z of Community Mental Health Practice.* USA: Singular Publishing Group.

Glick, R. L.., Berlin, J. S., Fishkind, A., and Zeller, S. (2008). *Emergency Psychiatry: Principles and Practice.* Canada: Lippincott Williams and Wilkins.

Holmes, D., Rudge, T., and Perron, A. (2013). *(Re)Thinking Violence in Health Care Settings: A Critical Approach.* Burlington, USA: Ashgate Publishing, Ltd.

Leather, P. (1999). Work-Related Violence: Assessment and Intervention. New York, NY: Routledge.

Shepherd, J. (2001) *Violence in Health Care Understanding, Preventing and Surviving Violence: A Practical Guide for Health Professionals.* Oxford: Oxford University press.

Wykes, T. (1994). *Violence and health care professionals.* London: Chapman & Hall.

Crisis Intervention and Prevention in Healthcare
Questions Chapter 5

1. Direct eye contact or nodding of head assures the patient that you are still interesting in the conversation

   True
   False

2. Reaching out your hand while talking to an aggressive person can seem like a threat

   True
   False

3. Abusive questions should not be ignored and should be answered

   True
   False

4. Healthcare professionals should practice self-control to avoid giving threats and showing that they are angry

   True
   False

5. Body language can be controlled to avoid stimulating anxiety

   True
   False

6. When conversing make lots of promises

   True
   False

7. Tension de-escalating can be achieved by attempting to solve the problem at the moment

   True
   False

8. Breathing exercises and relaxation can reduce tension

   True
   False

9. Healthcare professionals should not keep quiet or walk away if there are chances of engaging in an argument

   True
   False

10. You should call for back up if caught up in a crisis

    True
    False

11. Healthcare professionals should ensure the way to the exit is clear from obstruction

    True
    False

12. In strategies to avoid physical harm physical means are used as the first remedy

    True
    False

13. It is not appropriate to keep the legs apart and wide and leave the arms open when standing according to Bowie

True

False

14. An aggressor who is kicking can be difficult to handle

True

False

15. If one fall down while being attacked use the legs and feet to push away to prevent aggressive patient from further attacking

16. The most appropriate way to cause an aggressor to let go of the arm is to push the hand downward closest to the floor

True

False

17. The foot and hand can be used to block punches True/ False

18. When the hair is pulled make an effort to hold the aggressor's hands and direct them towards the head

True

False

19. Weapons should be hold with the right hand and the left hand is use to guard the eyes

True

False

20. If the aggressive patient is holding a gun escape by running in a straight line

True/ False

Chapter Six

Outline

1. Introduction.

2. Least restrictive measures

2.1.   Restraining techniques
2.2.   Psychological restraint
2.3.   Seclusion and Exclusion
2.4.   Mechanical restraint and Four-point restraint
2.5.   Restraining procedure
3. Appropriate use of medications as chemical

   restraints

3.1. Medication categories

   3.1.1. Butyrophenones
   3.1.2. Benzodiazepines
   3.1.3. Benzodiazepines and Butyrophenones
3.2. Atypical antipsychotics

3.3. Effects of chemical restraints

3.4. Administrations of chemical restraints

3.5. Implications of chemical restrain

4. Conclusion.

Crisis prevention and Intervention in healthcare
Introduction.

Restraining patients is a challenge because it has legal implications on the healthcare facility and the patient. The presence of a qualified healthcare professional is therefore considered necessary. Restraints prevent harm and can assist in the implementation of treatment. Guidelines and policies on restraints are provided by regulatory bodies to ensure that the restraint is only given when necessary and does not cause danger to the patient. To understand the concerns surrounding restraint, this chapter discusses restraining techniques and appropriate use of chemical restraints. Emphasis is placed on a restraint free environment.

2. Restraining techniques

Patients in crisis can be a threat to others and to self. The terms used in most mental health units are: Danger to Self (DTS) or Danger to others (DTO). Restraining entails restricting the arms, legs and strapping down the waist to reduce or contain mobility. Patients can be confined in hospital willingly or unwillingly. Restraint prevents a patient from moving their head, body, arms or legs freely. Items used to facilitate medical examination such as bandage are not considered restraints.

a. Least restrictive measures

Measures to restrain patients with assaultive behavior are carefully selected because restriction or seclusion could lead to negative outcomes if inapproriately implemented. Therefore, recommended measures should be least restrictive and steered towards specific results. Restraining techniques are recommended only when necessary. A patient can only be restrained following a physician's order. Advice for restraining by the healthcare professional should be accompanied by the length of time the assaultive person should be restrained. Observations should be made when the patient is restrained and recorded at regular intervals. Reviews can be made to assist the patients overcome their condition. Restraining is not used as a convenient way of containing the patient when healthcare professionals want to discipline the assaultive patient. A patient on restraints is usually on an every fifteen minute check.

Healthcare professionals should be aware of the body alignment when implementing least restriction to avoid body injuries. The patient should be able to change movement and exercise joints a bit. Body circulation is important to enable the body to continue functioning as Ballard and Rockett (2009, p. 34) mention.

b. Psychological restrain

Psychological restrain may precede chemical restrain and physical measures to restrain. Psychological restrain is given in the form of a program or a therapy. Activities are designed to meet the diverse situation of the assaultive behavior by withholding certain privileges. The privileges withdrawn do not include the basic needs. The patient being restrained will have access to shelter, clothing and food. Patients undergoing psychological restraint can interact with family, healthcare professionals and attorney. Psychological restraining is part of treatment which can be prescribed as a therapy.

c. Seclusion and Exclusion

Seclusion implies that a patient is placed in a separate area from others where the room is locked. When a patient asks to have own room that is open, it is not seclusion. A patient is not in seclusion if they are locked in a room because there is a quarantine to prevent spread of disease. The room where an aggressive patient is secluded is not locked if the patient is a child. The room is often watched and secured. Safe and soft items are availed for the aggressive patients to vent.

The objective of putting an aggressive patient in seclusion is not to cause harm, but to prevent the patient from becoming aggressive thereby reducing factors that encourage violence as Lewis and Ford (2000, p.34) discuss. Seclusion is given after the least restrictive policies have not been effective.

Exclusion takes place when a patient is moved from a one place to another restricted area. Patients with mental disorders who persistently do not cooperate with management intervention may be excluded from the other patients with mental disorders. Exclusion is different from seclusion because in exclusion the room is not locked while in seclusion the room is locked. Rooms for patients in exclusion are constantly monitored, since the assaultive patients are allowed to vent.

Seclusion and exclusion are a result of the physician's recommendations and should be limited. The healthcare professionals should remove dangerous items that could be used to cause harm from the room. Such items include clothing which can be used for strangling. Seclusion and exclusion cannot be administered on patients with substance overdose, and tendencies of self-harm.

d. Mechanical restraint and Four-point restraint

There are situations where the aggressive patient has acute violent behavior. The healthcare professional designs a mechanical restraint plan recognizing the imminent danger to self and others. The plan indicates how the restrain is to be done. Healthcare professionals trained to restrain aggressive patients use straps, wristlets, anklets, lockable buckles and muffs. The patient may be allowed certain movements at specified intervals. Mechanical restrain should be applied carefully to avoid harm and removed safely (Park et al, 2007, p. 13).

Four-point restrain is useful in emergency cases when containing a patient with mental disorder and violence. It is recommended after ways of deescalating violence are not sufficient.

When the de-escalating measures fail, measures could be put in place to reduce the chances of hurting the patient and healthcare professional while attempting to restrain them. Four point restraints can be done in the inpatient facility or the emergency room. The healthcare professional should make note of the rights of the patient.

There are dangerous positions for restraining the patient. For example, arms or legs should not be locked. Restrain where the face is facing down is currently considered illegal.

Inappropriate techniques cause the patient to experience pain which makes them struggle harder and subject them to unnecessary abuse (Ballard and Rockett 2009, p. 3).

e. Restraining procedure

Restraining a patient requires preparation to avoid incidents or injury. Johnson (2010, p. 182) suggests that, healthcare professionals with training should be prepared for emergencies and be willing to assist if required. Before attempting to restrain, obtain resources and the required number of people. Get the room ready before the patient is placed in seclusion or exclusion. Ask people by name to give a hand and inform them about the situation. Make a plan on how to approach the patient by assigning specific tasks to everyone. Reach the patient systematically and commit to play own part.

Appoint a leader who will give instructions when there is need to change the plan. The leader will assess the situation and make notes of the progress. Make an alternative plan incase events do not turn out as expected. The plan will entail a signal that there is success and a signal that there is failure. The leader will notify the team when efforts are fruitless and they should stop. There should be a clear way of stopping and exiting. Remind the team to avoid chocking or mishandling the assaultive patient. Be prepared to change the physical to chemical restrain if all efforts are not successful to prevent delayed intervention, especially when they continue to struggle after restrain. Do not be deceived by patients who suddenly calm down and comply to all instructions unexpectedly. This could be a sign of tiredness or in the worst case scenario the onset of an illness. Resist from screaming, but keep conversations going. Avoid warning healthcare professionals about what the patient might do because this may be taken as an idea by the assaultive patient.

3. Appropriate use of medications as chemical restraints

Chemical restraints are used to control behavior by administering medication. The medication is given according to individual's needs. The medication given to violent patients is short- term and is administered depending on the patient's history and circumstances. It is given on emergency to control behavior and to facilitate treatment (Mohr 2010, p. 5). Other chemical restrains are long- term and adjustments are made when the medicine is given to different patients. The long-term restraint is administered on a regular basis to smooth the progress and management of mental illness and behavioral disorders. After administration of any chemical restraint an assessment is done to establish underlying issues such as substance use, anxiety or mental illness (Tardiff, 1999, p. 237). Chemical restraints can be used concurrently with physical restraining techniques.

a. Medication categories

Chlorpromazine is a medication that has been used to sedate aggressive patients. However, Chlorpromazine's usefulness has been exceeded by adverse effects on tolerance; hence its use has been discontinued. Butyrophenones have been prescribed as an effective and safe medication for use in containing violent patients.

Butyrophenones have been successfully used together with benzodiazepines to restrain the assaultive behavior patient. Atypical antipsychotics are also used as chemical restrains as discussed by Halles and Frances (2005, p. 152).

i. Butyrophenones

Dropridol and haloperidol are Butyrophenones, which are also Neuroleptics. Dropridol is appropriate for agitation which causes sedation. Dropridol is a first line medication. Haloperidol is a tranquilizer for calming patients with violence. The medication is given in the form of injection. Dropridol and haloperidol are safe to use for those with substance abuse or overdose, but will require monitoring. Butyrophenones are also known as typical antipsychotics.

ii. Benzodiazepines

Benzodiazepines in the form of lorazepam and midazolam can also be used to cause tranquilization effects. Lorazepam is considered the best because of its short half-life, rapidness, inactive metabolites and effectiveness. Midazolam effects take a shorter time than Lorazepam, but is fast in effect and safe. Benzodiazepines are specifically recommended to patients with intoxication. Other assaultive patients can be given Benzodiazepines for control successfully.

iii. Benzodiazepines and Butyrophenones

A Combination of Benzodiazepines and Butyrophenones give superior effects than if used alone. One of the successful combinations is haloperidol and lorazepam. Patients respond to combined treatment faster than if given one treatment. Moreover, the side effects are minimal if a combined treatment is administered.

b. Atypical antipsychotics

Risperidone, ziprasidone and olanzapine are in the category of atypical antipsychotics. The medication is a recent development that corrects the negative effects of extrapyramidal symptoms. The medications have improved outcomes when compared with Butyrophenones. Atypical antipsychotics are tolerable by different groups of patients. The medication is specifically effective on patients with mental disorders in the short-term treatment.

c. Effects of chemical restraints

Chemical restraints may have effects such as depression of respiration and will require monitoring and proper adherence to policies to ensure safety. The chemical restraint is prescribed by the physician. Assessment is made on the patient's response on vital body organs and body response to the treatment.

Healthcare professionals should follow the recommended dosage according to the age of the person in crisis. Medication on pregnant and lactating mothers should be avoided. *Physical restraint* is not recommended for pregnant women because of injury to the spine when in the second and third trimester; hence *chemical restraints* are recommended. Neuroleptics should not be given to women who are pregnant or nursing. Medication should be discontinued if it causes negative effects (allergy) on

120

the patient. Patients with intoxication should not be given Neuroleptics, since it could cause seizures. Additional concern emerges since the medication could expose the fetus to abnormalities in development. Pregnant women are likely to develop respiratory issues. The fetus could have poor brain growth. Because there is no certainty if the chemical restrain could cause harm to the fetus, it is advisable to use minimal dosage.

Conversely, use of Butyrophenones can cause extrapyramidal symptoms which could cause blockage of the airway leading to mortality. Patients using chemical restraints may have disturbed mental conditions, high blood pressure, rigid muscles and hyperthermia. The conduct of the patient can be disturbed because of sedation. Benzodiazepine causes patients to become sedated, nauseated and confused. Patients who have taken alcohol are at risk of getting respiratory depression if they are given Benzodiazepines (Rund et al, 2006, p. 318).

According to Mion (2008, p. 422), the healthcare professional should avoid pitfalls that are associated with failure to monitor signs of sedation. Avoid misdiagnosis of agitation and increased anxiety. The nurse should be able to recognize adverse effects of medication on time.

d. Administrations of chemical restraints

The desired use for the chemical restrains owes to the fact that the effect is rapid and there seems to be reduced side effects. Giving the medication orally is preferred to intramuscular administration.

Medication is given using intramuscular means if they fail to cooperate and if there is imminent danger. Patients offered oral medication before intramuscular injection tend to trust the healthcare professionals which enable the delivery of efficient service.

This is because the patient gains internal form of control as opposed to external control from the healthcare professional. Dissolving formulas and oral concentrated are preferred to the tablets. Tablets are discouraged because patients can hide them in the mouth and fail to swallow. In mental health, it is called 'cheeking' medications.

Additionally, tablets take a long time to begin action when compared to dissolving formulas and intramuscular medication. Intravenous is the most preferred because it has the highest score in commencement of action. Therefore, intramuscular or intravenous medication is the most appropriate in emergencies. Tablets are given in the long-term treatment. Obtaining the intramuscular and intravenous medication is more difficult than accessing tablets. Medications administered orally are introduced before the intramuscular and intravenous medication (Rund et al, 2006, p. 321).

e. Implications of chemical restraint

Legal implications should be considered when a patient is restrained. Different governments have authorized and others illegalized restraining techniques and use of chemical restrain, by implementing policies and giving guidelines. While some may perceive chemical restrain as a medication, other states do not advocate for it because of its side effects. Healthcare professionals would have to make professional judgment before choosing the chemical restraint because the patient has a right to and can make a complaint. The healthcare professional should obtain an informed consent from the patient and explain the treatment if they are of sound mind. As a result, the patient can reject or accept medication for restrain if they understand the course of treatment. If the patient is incompetent and poses immediate danger, the healthcare professional can perform chemical restraints without consent. In this case, the consent form signed during the admission that allows the physicians and nurses to make decisions for the patient in emergency would cover the emergency consent not obtained. Otherwise, the healthcare professional should allow the patient make a decision to avoid charges of false imprisonment.

A restrain free environment is emphasized to prevent the negative effects of restrain. Patients under restrain have been found to suffer injuries from falls, broken bones, impaired circulation, incontinence, social isolation and depression. Some patients have committed suicide with available pieces of cloths and others injured from attempting to escape (Center for Ethics and Human Rights, 2012, p. 2). Nurses should recognize the early signs of assaultive behavior and utilize verbal de-escalation techniques to prevent the patient from rising to the stage of crisis. Early de-escalation techniques are very important and need to be applied to ensure a restrain free environment. I have worked in a mental health facility where our restraining actions were very minimal because de-escalation techniques where often used. I have also worked in another mental health facility where take-down was a daily routine. The difference between high rate and low rate of restraining cases lies heavily on how the healthcare professionals treat patients. The importance of early recognition of the assault cycle and verbal de-escalation cannot be over-emphasized.

4. Conclusion.

Restraining is done to prevent harm on patient and others. It sometimes enables healthcare professionals treat and control behavior of patient. Restraining techniques often implemented consist of least restrictive measures, psychological, seclusion and exclusion, mechanical and four-point restraint.

The strategies protect the rights of patients and are based on individual needs. Restraining is recommended and implemented by healthcare professionals who monitor the progress and give recommendation. Restraint are administered and removed safely by trained healthcare professionals. Regulatory bodies recommend less restraining procedures, time limits and keeping of a record.

Chemical restraints are used if other restraining techniques prove futile. Medications that are used include: Benzodiazepines (lorazepam, midazolam), Butyrophenones (dropridol, haloperidol), and atypical antipsychotics (ziprasidone, risperidone, olanzapine).

The medications sedate the patient to control behavior. Although the chemical restraints are safe to use, they can cause effects such as depression, hyperthermia, mental conditions, and rigid muscles or affect vital organs; hence the patient should be monitored. Chemical restraints are best administered in the form of dissolving formulas and oral concentrated or intramuscular or intravenous injection.

The healthcare professional should be aware of the legal implications to avoid pitfalls. A restrain free environment is suggested since it limits the number of injuries and other disadvantages associated with restraints.

References

Ballard, B. and Rockett, J. (2009). *Restraint & Handling for Veterinary Technicians &   Assistants.* United States: Delmar Cengage Learning.

Center for Ethics and Human Rights (2012). *Reduction of Patient Restraint and Seclusion in Health Care Settings.* Action Report.

Halles, R. and Frances, A. (2005) *Psychiatry Update: The American Psychiatric Association   Annual Review.* United States: The American Psychiatric Association.

Johnson, M. (2010). Violence and restraint reduction efforts on inpatient psychiatric units. *Issues in Mental Health Nursing,* 31, 181–187.

Lewis, E., and Ford, J. (2000). *Hostile Ground: Defusing and Restraining Violent Behavior and   Physical Assaults.* Paladin Press

Mion, L. (2008). Physical restraint in critical care settings. *Geriatric Nursing,* 29 (6), 421–423.

Mitzel, K., and Votolato, N. (2006). The use of intramuscular benzodiazepines and antipsychotic agents in the treatment of acute agitation or violence in the emergency department. *Journal of Emergency Medicine,* 31, (3),317-324.

Mohr, W. K. (2010). Restraints and the code of ethics: An uneasy fit. *Archives of Psychiatric Nursing,* 24(1), 3–14.

Park, M., Hsiao-Chen Tang, J., Adams, S., & Titler, M. (2007). Evidence-based guideline: Changing the practice of physical restraint use in acute care. *Journal of Gerontological*

Nursing, 33(2), 9–16.

Rund, D. A., Ewing, J., Tardiff, K. (1999). *Medical Management of the Violent Patient: Clinical Assessment and Therapy (Medical Psychiatry Series).* CRC Press.

Crisis Intervention and Prevention in Healthcare
Questions Chapter 6

1. Patients can be confined in hospital willingly or unwillingly

   True
   False

2. A bandage is considered to be a restraint

   True
   False

3. Restraining is a convenient way of containing a patient when healthcare professionals want to discipline the assaultive patient

   True
   False

4. Psychological restrain is given in the form of a program or therapy

   True
   False

5. Seclusion implies that a patient is locked in a room because there is a quarantine to prevent the spread of disease

   True
   False

6. Exclusion means the room is not locked

   True
   False

7. Seclusion and exclusion should be administered on patients with substance overdose and is suicidal

    True
    False

8. Mechanical restrain should be applied carefully to avoid harm

    True
    False

9. Four-point restrain is useful in emergency cases to contain patient with mental disorder ad violence

    True
    False

10. Four-point restrain can only be used in the inpatient facility

    True
    False

11. Arms and legs should be locked when restraining a patient

    True
    False

12. Team members should be reminded to avoid choking and mishandling the assaultive patient

    True
    False

13. Chemical restraints is given to violent patient according to their needs

    True

False

14. Long-term restrain is administered on a regular basis to smooth the progress and manages of mental illness and behavioral disorders

True
False

15. _____ is a medication that has been used to sedate aggressive patients

   A. Risiperidone

   B. Haloperidol

   C. Chlorpromazine

16. Which of the following are also used as chemical restrains

   A. Atypical antipsychotics

   B. Benzodiazepines

   C. Haloperidol

17. Which of the following medication is appropriate for agitation which causes sedation

   A. Haloperidol

   B. Dropridol

   C. Tylenol

18. _____ is used as a tranquilizer for calming patients with violence

   A. Haloperidol

   B. Midol

   C. Benadryl

19. Which of the following are in the category of atypical antipsychotics

   A. Risperidon, ziprasidone

   B. Olanzapine

   C. All of the above

20. Neuroleptics is safe to give to women when they are pregnant

   True
   False

Chapter Seven

Crisis Prevention and Intervention.
Emergency Preparedness for Healthcare Facilities.

Outline

1. Introduction

2. Earthquake

3. Terrorism

4. Carbon Monoxide poisoning

5. Hurricane

6. Floods

7. Tornadoes

8. Tsunami

9. Volcanoes

10. Landslides

Crisis Prevention & Intervention
(Emergency Preparedness for Healthcare Facilities)

Introduction

This chapter would discuss the emergency preparedness that hospital communities should observe during a certain suspected occurrence of a disaster. First, it is pertinent to note that disaster usually comes in all sizes and shapes; it can be either fabricated or natural. Notably, the following are some of the suspected disasters that need attention by the whole hospital community. Suspected calamities are: the earthquake, landslide, hurricanes, floods, Tornadoes, terrorism, volcanoes, tsunami, what to do if someone attacks the hospital with a weapon and lastly carbon Monoxide poisoning. It is advisable that since a hospital is working as a team, then the fight and preparedness here should also be initiated as a team.

Outside the hospital workers and patients, when people are anticipating for an outbreak of any kind of disaster that may range from an earthquake, a disease, terrorism, and/or fire, hospitals are always on a high alert in view of combating the outbreak. This happens because if any of these outbreaks eventually occurs, those who become victims always require medical attention (Rout & Rout, 2002). Thus, putting in place a substantial medical system for attending any emergencies is congruent at such times.

In emergency preparedness, medical professionals as well as other hospital staff set themselves in place in order to handle any cases that may require medical attention. In view of bracing for such events, there are procedures and protocols that the concerned professionals follow (Veenema, 2007).They are not complex, but consistent and ensure that the safety of humans comes first. This chapter will seek to discuss emergency preparedness for healthcare providers by providing ten different areas where hospitals should exhibit emergency preparedness.

Earthquake

It is vital to raise concern over earthquake occurrence in the hospital. Earthquake is natural and often, hard to identify the direction to which it is originating from without some machinery assistance. Therefore, it is advisable for the hospital management to be well equipped with several kits that can last over seventy-two hours after the occurrence of the real incidence. Some of the kits are the ponchos, radios for communication and networking, food rations and flashlights just to sample but a few. Again, it is important for the hospital management to acknowledge the vitality of the emergency systems that will aid in notifications. Further, it will be awesome if the hospital is safe-guarded with earthquake safety measures. Frames and foundations of the building should be reinforced to resist earthquake.

Analysts advise that whenever there is an earthquake, people should always drop, cover, and hold on. In real terms, this means that one should first look for a place to drop and cover him or herself when the earth starts trembling. This in effect reduces the chances of any person falling casualty of such natural disasters. However, noting that the occurrence of such natural disasters requires that the inception of certain measures is substantial (Veenema, 2007). This means that if a certain area requires helping people survive an earthquake and thereafter reduce its health impacts, they must first of all prepare, come up with a plan, and practice. Whenever earthquakes occur, loss of lives and properties accompanied by panic is rampant. In addition, hospitals and other healthcare facilities resolve to help reduce the impacts that result from such natural disasters (Rout & Rout, 2002). Overly, earthquakes and other natural disasters tend to send a series of panic and havoc among the proclaimed victims. As such, analysts have come to consider these attacks as some of the major contributors of losses suffered during the event of an earthquake.

Far in advance, surveys show that whenever weather professionals forecast any possibility of a threatening earthquake, medical professionals and hospital staff wander up and down in search of ways of combating the repercussions.

Prospects show that when an earthquake is about to occur, medical professionals and hospital staff gather emergency supplies (Veenema, 2007). This means that in order to be in a position to combat the impacts of such natural disaster, the concerned professionals must get down in search of the necessary emergency supplies that can help either reduce or stop the effects of an earthquake. After that, hospital professionals identify and work tirelessly with the aim of reducing the risks within the places affected. Identifying the possible areas of destruction is crucial as it helps reduce the amount of lives or properties that could perish in the face of an earthquake (Rout & Rout, 2002). What follows these steps is the aspect of practicing the measures to take during and at the end of an earthquake. Medical professionals ascertain that practicing what to do at the time of an earthquake and after can help people remain healthy and safe (Clements, 2009). One can never over emphasize the importance of earthquake drills. Practice! Practice!! Practice!!!

Fire

What starts as a simple spark can result to an uncontrollable fire in less than thirty seconds. Prospects indicate that fire spreads very easily and requires just a few seconds to become what fire extinguishers and related experts otherwise term as risky and uncontrollable.

Nevertheless, emergency preparedness for fire with regard to hospital professionals is always significant (Reilly & Markenson, 2011).

It comes to such a situation when hospitals' professionals seek to bring together the necessary equipment that can help reduce the consequences of a fire outbreak.

Under these circumstances, the level of readiness is very important as it helps determine the extent at which the hospital professionals will react to a fire outbreak. Since fire can shake a whole hospital, it is always vital for doctors and other assisting personnel to equip themselves with the general elements of managing an emergency (Hogan & Burstein, 2007). In an event of fire, hospital professionals prepare themselves in view of combating this epidemic by setting up an incident command system, which facilitates the integration of the community emergency planning commonly forwarded by the available groups. Hospital professionals also equip themselves with decontamination materials in the wake of a fire outbreak (Rosdahl & Kowalski, 2008).

Decontamination is a part of the emergency preparedness procedures that are employed at any given time when fire incidents are on the rise. It is important to indicate that even though medical professionals should always seek to avail preparedness, materials for an emergency in position in case of a fire outbreak, turning for other measures is even more substantial (Reilly & Markenson, 2011).

Specialists in the fire department maintain that evacuation is indeed a congruent strategy that hospital professionals should always consider in an event of fire as it ensures safety and hospital expenditures in the long run.

Given that these emergency preparedness measures may help reduce the impacts of a fire outbreak, turning around for disaster recovery procedures is preliminary (Clements, 2009).

It helps restore those affected by the fire tragedy to their previous status but this happens in places where such a move is possible.

Terrorism

Documented evidence states that disasters may be natural while others are man-made. Terrorism is an example of artificial disaster that may cause people loss of their lives and in other cases, loss, or destruction of their properties (Ciottone, 2006). In whichever case, terrorism does not result into anything productive but rather diminishes any feeling of freedom and security within and outside the said territory.

Take a look at the September 9/11 terrorist attacks; it is notable that both the American citizens and the outside world felt threatened security wise (Veenema, 2007).

As a result, the government, with the support of other concerned organizations resolved to form such groups like the Local Emergency Planning Committees, which supports hospital professionals in combating terrorism activities.

It is therefore deducible that one way in which hospital professionals prepare for terrorist emergencies is via forming negotiation and support committees that help facilitate the delivery of services to the affected individuals (Hogan & Burstein, 2007).

There may be an incident where someone comes in to attack the hospital with a weapon. Here, it is advisable that both patients and hospital officials should make a highway where some individuals can escape.

In addition, the alarm system should be in place and in good condition, which will alert the security officers on the attack immediately.

At times, terrorist activities may include holding innocent citizens hostage, shooting and wounding individuals, and/or releasing hazardous gases into an enclosed building. Under these circumstances, the lives of many people are always at stake, a situation that calls for emergency preparedness in not only hospitals but also in security agencies (Rosdahl & Kowalski, 2008). Of late, terrorist and other related criminal activities have skyrocketed and the available means of combating their consequences are being diversified. Hospital professionals equip themselves with emergency handling facilities such as masks and gloves if they are up against hazardous gases.

The increased rate of potential attacks by the terrorist directs the consequence and unique burden on Medical personnel. Therefore, it is the responsibility of the hospital management to prepare in advance for the fight against such act.

Thus, the hospital officials have the mandate to implement policies that will protect health care personnel during the time when they will be attending to the victims. Therefore, it is pertinent to have ambulance in standby to evacuate some patients to other hospitals, order extra medical supplies and make arrangements for security personnel.

The terrorists may shoot and injure their victims making it hard for the hospital professionals to just sit and wait for the final decision.

Carbon Monoxide poisoning

Chemical analysis shows that carbon monoxide is simply a gas that is colorless and odorless but very poisonous when it reaches its maximum and can lead to a sudden death due to the body's lack of oxygen.

Overly, experts in gaseous response propose that carbon monoxide which emanates from motor vehicles, gas powered generators, fire, power washers, boats, charcoal grill, and other gas powered equipment can cause death when in sufficient supply within the ambient air (Ciottone, 2006).

Research findings suggest that the most at risk populations consist of the elderly, babies, infants, and people who suffer from chronic respiratory illnesses, anemia, and/or heart diseases (Landesman, 2005). In an event of carbon monoxide poisoning, hospital professionals should equip themselves with oxygen gas and resolve to consider carrying out hyperbaric oxygen therapy (HBO).

Educational scores in carbon monoxide positioning and related studies suggest that oxygen gas is a substantial remedy against carbon monoxide poisoning mainly because it relieves the patient of hypoxemia as it helps supply the heart with adequate oxygen capable of pumping blood to the other parts of the body (Veenema, 2007)

Aside from oxygen, healthcare professionals should also exhibit emergency preparedness in an event when a patient is brought in with Carbon Monoxide level above or between 25 and 30 percent.

In such circumstances, a patient may lose his or her life to cardiac involvement, neurological impairment, and/or prolonged unconsciousness (Hogan & Burstein, 2007). Generally, when healthcare professionals carry out a hyperbaric oxygen therapy and diagnose a patient with severe acidosis, cardiac disease, or transient unconsciousness, they should always consider the matter as an emergency case as the patient may die from these signs (Clements, 2009).

Just as clinicians suggest, harmful gases such as carbon monoxide pose significant challenges to people's livelihoods and should always be treated with much haste as they cannot only impair the health of the victim, but also lead to the consequent death of the affected person (Reilly & Markenson, 2011). Therefore, considering carbon monoxide poisoning as an emergency cannot be over-emphasized. The management team should ensure that there is proper installation of the carbon monoxide alarms, which can alert the concern to responsible individuals audibly. The hospitals should have a professional checker of all burning appliances. It is not wise to be using oven or range to assist in heating the hospitals. Charcoal burning in hospital should be out of bounds. Another caution is that cars should not be left running since; this will not supply required air in the milieu. Hospitals should develop extra decontamination rooms since it is not likely that pre-hospital personnel will manage to control all the contamination issues, the above will prevent hypothermia.

For seriously affected patients, application of chest radiography is recommendable particularly those showing signs of cardiopulmonary failure and lack of consciousness as they may require emergency services more than others may.

Hurricane

A Cyclone or a typhoon or other tropical storms could occur. Hospitals and healthcare professionals should at all times consider a hurricane to be a disaster that requires emergency attention and prepare for them majorly because they lead to the destruction of homes, industrial outlets, and social supplies such as water, electricity, and food (Rosdahl & Kowalski, 2008).

A hurricane is another disaster that needs thorough preparedness. For any hospitals to run effectively without worries of the severity of the hurricane, it is important that the following issues be put in place: Back-up generators are required to prevent black out condition. Hospital structures should be hardened and category five windows hurricane resistance put in place. Fuel tanks for the back-up generators should be available.

In the event of a hurricane, strong winds blow. They tend to destroy power lines causing a total blackout, which leads to people living in particular area being cut off from the outside world, as they cannot watch the news or receive any supplies.

There could also be loss of lives as a hurricane destroys buildings, trapping those inside and making it hard for them to survive without the essentials of humans.

With this respect, considering a hurricane to be a natural disaster that requires emergent attention is crucial for healthcare professionals as it can help save lives of the affected by providing them with the necessary medical attention capable of sustaining their lives (Landesman, 2005). Hurricanes can trap patients and medical professionals in the facility without the ability of getting out, and that is if they are alive.

Hurricanes cause havoc and panic over many people and this may trigger health complications within people who suffer from coronary and other heart diseases. For such people to survive, they require emergency medical attention, which only medically trained personnel, can provide (Ciottone, 2006).

This means that hospitals and healthcare professionals should always treat hurricane as an emergency case so that they can resolve to provide either medical attention to people brought to them with such complications or those they choose to rescue (Clements, 2009).

Further, healthcare providers should always consider hurricane as an emergency issue since it requires people to evacuate their places of residence. In an event of evacuation, healthcare professionals can offer many medical related services to those evacuating considering the situation, as an emergency. Hurricanes trigger a number of issues such as diseases and infections as well as injuries since the heavy winds tend to lead to falling trees and buildings (Wolfson, Hendey, & Harwood-Nuss, 2010).

Floods

Another natural disaster is the flood. It is worthy to note that floods being a natural disaster calls for preparedness immediately when any sign is noted to avoid loss of life. Some of the preparedness process is that, it is important that emergency teams be available so that they bear mandate of pumping excess water out of the building. Plans are supposed to be in place for the relocation of the patients in the intensive care unit, those on hemodialysis and those who are in ventilators. If that is not enough, the hospital management should create a route where, during the flood, the responsible team should access the basement and do the required repair.

Further, it is required that safe route to be improvised so the patients and other individuals can run to a nearby shelter, for instance a raised pucca house. Emergency kits should be accessible. The emergency kits must have; the torch, portable radio and spare battery. Fresh water stocks, candle, dry food and match boxes. It is important to have polythene bags, waterproof that can act as valuables and clothing bamboo stick and umbrellas. Lastly, the first aid kit should have strong ropes that will assist in tying and manuals.

In relation to the community, healthcare professionals should prepare for floods. Agreeably, floods cause diseases, infections, and other malicious ailments that cause deaths and loss of properties (Rosdahl & Kowalski, 2008).

Buildings collapse and structured centers fall apart when floods occur and this is the major reason as to why healthcare professionals should always consider floods as an emergency at all times. This means that healthcare professionals should exhibit preparedness at an event of floods since they result in diseases such as cholera and infections such as typhoid. In tropical regions, floods cause other diseases like malaria since mosquitoes breed in such zones making it hard for the residents to survive in such conditions (Veenema, 2007). Healthcare professionals should be fully prepared in an event of flood since floods bring about contaminations, which require immunization and treatment.

When floods fill houses and other settlement buildings, chances of those buildings collapsing are always high. In case they collapse, those present fall victims and sustain major injuries that always require medical attention. Truthfully, not all personnel involved in evacuation when there are floods are capable of handling an influx of patients with injuries (Clements, 2009). This means that if healthcare professionals consider floods as an emergency, it becomes easier to combat the impacts of such natural disasters. Healthcare providers should therefore find floods to be tormenting and exhibit preparedness in the event of such incidences in order to help reduce the damages that may result from them (Landesman, 2005). Apparently, floods raise concerns over sanitation cases and in many incidents, the affected places always have a large number of people who suffer from health complications after consuming contaminated foods. When such situations occur, people tend to require urgent medical attention, which without the help of qualified medical personnel, events can always turn out to be devastating (Hogan & Burstein, 2007). In summary, when floods occur, healthcare professionals should exhibit preparedness, as they are part of the panel that can help save lives through various attempts.

Tornadoes

A tornado is another disaster that needs a hospital to be well prepared in any case it occurs. Since it is a violent wind, called whirlwinds and it usually crosses the land in a narrow path, it can cause death and so it needs correct measures to be put in place.

Here, the required preparedness is as follows; the vulnerable parties like patients should be protected by every practical and feasible means available. Some of this practice are blinding and closing the windows. Patients should be covered with blankets and nursing personnel are supposed to move patients to the hallways. All individuals should move to the interior, the hospital management should make the security available.

Any person at the site, who does not have security officers, should be designated as a spotter. When people become aware of a possible occurrence of a tornado and immediately seek ways of evading it, the damage caused by such natural disasters can be greatly reduced.

Adhering to tornado warnings and implications can help save many lives as the set emergency evacuation and combating policies are always the best remedy for these disasters (Wolfson, Hendey, & Harwood-Nuss, 2010).

An ongoing tornado poses serious challenges and risks to people's lives as they carry with them heavily blown objects and risk killing people through falling or flying objects as the winds are always fast and strong. After a tornado, those wreckages that remain behind present additional risks to people's lives as they can result in risky injuries. Specialists maintain that nothing can be done in order to prevent the occurrence of a tornado but taking the necessary actions that can help combat the risks that a tornado poses is essential (Rosdahl & Kowalski, 2008). Just as in the case of other natural disasters, tornadoes break power lines, electrical systems, and gas lines and can cause huge explosions or electrocution.

Healthcare professionals should exhibit preparedness in an event of a tornado since the challenges it poses are great in depth. Systemically, a wave of a tornado can leave hundreds of people dead and properties worth millions of dollars destroyed.

According to American Medical Association (AMA), tornadoes cause injuries to the people living within the affected areas, which may result from an impact caused by a falling tornado. During rescue attempts, the involved persons can barely make it out the area without an injury (Clements, 2009).

For example, during the rescue attempts of the tornado that took place in Marion, Illinois indicated that 50 percent of all the recorded injuries occurred during the rescue. People who walk among the debris may also sustain serious injuries as well as those entering damaged buildings (Trufanov, Rossodivita, & Guidotti, 2010). Research shows that when such a disaster occurs, people suffer many complications that require medical attention and therefore healthcare professionals should consider a tornado an emergency issue and resonate to set up an emergency preparedness platform (Reilly & Markenson, 2011).

Tsunami

When a tsunami takes place, it is likely that many people will either suffer from multiple health issues or lose their lives in the process.

In the occurrence of the tsunami, several practices should be carried out, for instance hospitals should carry out the pre-event preparedness, triage and patient evacuation. It is pertinent to carry out recognition of the hospital and secondary transfer, discharge where necessary and reduction of the admission procedures. Last, at this point, it is pertinent for the hospital management to reinforce the medical system to be well trusted.

During and after a tsunami is a very vibrant time for healthcare professionals as the press puts them in everyone's view, as they are the number one respondents of such disasters (Landesman, 2005). The most tormenting moments for a healthcare provider is the period after a tsunami occurs.

This is so because once the involved personnel rescue survivors, the concerned healthcare professionals and the government officials put their primary apprehension to clean water for drinking, shelter, and food as well as medical support for those who suffer injuries. This is a clear indication that healthcare professionals should always exhibit preparedness at a time of tsunami since their expertise is crucial and can help reduce damage and save many lives (Wolfson, Hendey, & Harwood-Nuss, 2010). Without a doubt, tsunamis lead to loss of shelter hence exposing the survivors to insects and heat among many other environmental risks (Rosdahl & Kowalski, 2008). Majority of the deaths that occur during and after a tsunami are caused by many hazards such as drowning.

Lately, researchers have come to conclude that injuries result from people being thrown by water into debris, which include but not limited to houses, stationary items, and trees (Clements, 2009). During these moments, people may sustain injuries such as head injuries and broken limbs that commonly result from physical impacts when water washes the caught victims into debris. Indeed, tsunamis are health and life risks and they can result to losses and destruction of either of the said items. Hence, it is agreeable to mention that healthcare professionals and other hospital staff should always exhibit preparedness during and after a tsunami (Reilly & Markenson, 2011). Combating the physical outcomes of a tsunami can prove to be daunting given that it causes masses of injuries that require immediate medical attention and within populated areas, a tsunami can alter a whole country's budget since the affected persons require not only safe food and clean drinking water, but also need new shelters (Wolfson, Hendey, & Harwood-Nuss, 2010).

Volcanoes

These natural phenomena occur in specific areas and specialists propagate that people have as many ways as there are of avoiding fallings victims of dangers that come along with a volcano eruption.

Profoundly, volcanoes can end up producing such things like flashfloods, toxic gases, ash, and fast moving flows of things like hot gases and other substances termed by geologists as pyroclastic flows (Rosdahl & Kowalski, 2008). Moreover, a volcano eruption can result to emission of hot water flashfloods and some debris otherwise referred to as lahars. The emergency plan should include the following; hazardous zones should be identified and marked, valuable property should be in register, safe refuge zones should be identified, so that hospital population can be evacuated if there are dangerous eruptions. Additionally, evacuations routes should be identified, assembly point be marked, this will help those who are waiting for transportation to the next safe hospital to converge easily. Means of transport should be identified, presence of the alert procedures, still during evacuation, it is vital for health care personnel to improvise mobile treatment. Correct communications should be put in place. It is vital to establish a good system for updates.

Always, it is important to pay attention to volcano warnings and is necessary to take the necessary measures in order to avoid any risks that may result from a volcano when it erupts. Undoubtedly, volcano eruption is a natural disaster that refutes mayhem upon those affected and stating that it requires healthcare professionals and other hospital attendants to exhibit preparedness is crucial (Hogan & Burstein, 2007). Disasters such as a volcano eruption, wildfire, and other public health emergencies can cause long lasting trauma that can reverberate with not only those affected but also those not directly affected.

Medical organizations, healthcare providers, and other hospital staff should exhibit emergency medical preparedness in an event of a volcanic eruption since the outcomes of such an event can result in heart breaking events in the lives of those involved in either way (Landesman, 2005). Presence of medical personnel in a case where there has occurred a volcano eruption can have outstanding effects on all sides. This is consequential because they help provide general strategies that promote mental health stability among those mentally traumatized (Trufanov, Rossodivita, & Guidotti, 2010). Center for disease and control works round the clock to help identify and track down any environmental hazards, health risks, and life threatening happenings that it then documents and calls for the necessary measures. Data provided by CDC expounds that a volcano dilapidates the essence of life wellness and revamps the aspect of life threatening events (Wolfson, Hendey, & Harwood-Nuss, 2010).

Based on such arguments, healthcare professionals in association with any other medical personnel should take the issue of volcano eruptions as a disaster that requires emergent attention and exhibit preparedness using the necessary means possible.

Landslides

Succinctly, landslides and/or mudslides happen when masses of earth parts, rocks, or debris fall down a slope making the neighboring parts sink together with the affected place. Mudslides otherwise termed as debris flows are the most rampant types of fast moving landslides and tend to flow in specific channels (Clements, 2009).

Research findings point out that a landslide occurs when there is a disturbance within the natural stability of a given slope. Unlike fabricated disasters, landslides can come along with earthquakes, volcanic eruptions, heavy droughts, and/or rains (Wolfson, Hendey, & Harwood-Nuss, 2010). Since landslides result from other formations such as when water develops or accumulates rapidly on a ground causing a surge in water saturation on a rock, debris, or earth, it leads to an outbreak of diseases. Further, it gives rise to diseases and other infections that are hazardous to human lives (Rosdahl & Kowalski, 2008). For all what is worth, healthcare providers should show emergency preparedness for a landslide since it poses life-threatening effects onto the involved individuals.

Landslide is an uncommon disaster that needs emergency preparedness. Here, it is pertinent for hospital management to stay awake and alert.

This is because it is evident that much debris usually occurs during nighttime. Therefore, alertness will save many lives if landslides will actually occur. Another important factor is that the hospital management should arrange for alternative places for evacuation, alert the security and rescue teams, and ensure phones and any other communication devices are in order.

Conclusion

In conclusion, after addressing those several issues that need emergency preparedness, I believe that disaster preparedness is well known to hospital personnel.

Therefore, it is important for hospitals to revise their plans on how to cover additional varieties of disasters that have in one way or another stuck at the roadblock. Here, a fact to put into consideration is to check if institutions are on the right track in their arrangement for the emergency preparedness.

Further, it is pertinent for the hospital management to involve all the departments. By doing that, it will be possible for the all voices to converge in one language and be heard. Another notable point is that, individuals should engage in not only practice but also training so that disaster management communication between the hospital and the community is effective. Hence, everyone will have open minds and that when disaster strikes, they will be well prepared and will face it courageously and positively.

As described above, natural disasters such as wildfire, volcano eruptions, hurricanes, landslides, tornadoes, and tsunamis among others can lead to total destruction of properties on one end (Trufanov, Rossodivita, & Guidotti, 2010) and on the other part, they can lead to many deaths if not combated at the relevant time.

This happens to be one of the most important reasons as to why healthcare professionals, emergency personnel, and other care providers should consider such events as emergent and requiring immediate attention (Landesman, 2005).

Therefore, they should always exhibit preparedness as failure to be ready for such emergencies can resolve to produce the largest casualties possible.

This chapter has provided an emergency preparedness insight for healthcare providers by giving different areas where a hospital should exhibit emergency preparedness.

References

Ciottone, G. R. (2006). *Disaster medicine*. Philadelphia: Elsevier Mosby.

Clements, B. (2009). *Disasters and public health: Planning and response*. Amsterdam: Butterworth-Heinemann/Elsevier.

Hogan, D. E. & Burstein, J. L. (2007). *Disaster medicine*. Philadelphia: Wolters Kluwer.

Landesman, L. Y. (2005). *Public health management of disasters: The practice guide*. Washington, DC: American Public Health Association.

Reilly, M. J. & Markenson, D. S. (2011). *Health care emergency management: Principles and practice*. Sudbury, Mass: Jones and Bartlett Learning.

Rosdahl, C. B. & Kowalski, M. T. (2008). *Textbook of basic nursing*. Philadelphia: Lippincott Williams & Wilkins.

Rout, U. & Rout, J. K. (2002). *Stress management for primary health care professionals*. New York: Kluwer Academic/Plenum.

Trufanov, A., Rossodivita, A., & Guidotti, M. (2010). *Pandemics and bioterrorism: Transdisciplinary information sharing for decision-making against biological threats*. Amsterdam: IOS Press.

Veenema, T. G. (2007). *Disaster nursing and emergency preparedness: For chemical, biological, and radiological terrorism and other hazards*. New York: Springer Pub.

Wolfson, A. B., Hendey, G. W., & Harwood-Nuss, A. (2010). *Harwood-Nuss' clinical practice of emergency medicine*. Philadelphia, PA: Lippincott Williams & Wilkins.

Crisis Intervention and Prevention in Healthcare
Questions Chapter 7

1. Whenever earthquakes occur loss of lives and properties accompanied by panic is rampant

   True
   False

2. Medical professionals ascertain that practicing what to do at the time of and after an earthquake can help people remain healthy and safe

   True
   False

3. The level of readiness is not important to help determine the extent at which the hospital professionals will react to a fire outbreak

   True
   False

4. _____ is a part of hospital emergency preparedness procedures that may employ at any given time when fire incidents are in a rise

   A. Decontamination

   B. Contamination

   C. Disinfectant

5. Which of the following is an example of artificial disaster that may cause people loss of their lives

A. Tsunami

B. Tornado

C. Terrorism

6. Hospital professionals should not equip themselves with emergency handling facilities such as gloves and masks if they are up against hazardous gases

   True
   False

7. _____ is a colorless, odorless, poisonous gas

   A. Oxygen

   B. Carbon monoxide

   C. Hydrogen

8. Carbon monoxide can emanate from which of the following

   A. Boats

   B. Charcoal grills

   C. Fire

   D. All of the above

9. Healthcare professionals should always consider hurricanes as emergencies and prepare for them

   True

False

10. Hurricanes cause havoc and panic which may trigger health complications among people who suffer from coronary diseases

   True
   False

11. Floods cause diseases, infections and other ailments that cause death and loss of properties

   True
   False

12. During the rescue attempts of the tornado that took place in Marion, Illinois 50% of all the injuries occurred before the rescue

   True
   False

13. The most tormenting moments for a healthcare provider is the period after a _____ occurs

   A. Tsunami

   B. Earthquake

   C. Hurricane

14. _____ can produce things like toxic gases, ash and flash floods

   A. Hurricane

   B. Tornadoes

C. Volcanoes

15. Which of the following organization work around the clock to identify and track environmental hazards and health risks

A. American Medical Association (AMA)

B. Center for Disease Control (CDC)

C. Federal Trade Commission (FTC)

16. _____ happen when masses of earth parts, rocks or debris fall down a slope

A. Landslide

B. Land glide

C. Land slope

17. Which of the following disasters one should always drop, cover and hold on

A. Hurricane

B. Fire

C. Earthquake

18. Hospital level of readiness is only important in some disasters not all

True
False

19. The most at risk populations for carbon monoxide consist of which of the following

A. Babies

B. Elderly

C. People who suffer from chronic respiratory illness

D. All of the above

20. Which of the following is not a natural disaster

A. Hurricane

B. You setting someone's car on fire

C. tornadoes

Miscellaneous Review Questions

1)   …................ is a violent behavior against another individual?
A Negligence
B Assaultive behavior
C Invasion of privacy
D Trauma

2) Some of the symptoms of assaultive behavior include the following, except
A Hand washing
B Slamming of doors
C Clenching of jaws
D Easily startled

3) Aggressive behavior is precipitated by the following except
A Smiling

B Prejudices
C Hostility
D Frustrations

4) Which of the following health conditions is not linked with aggressive behaviors
A Acute intoxication
B Myasthenia gravis
C Acute paranoid psychosis
D Antisocial personality disorder

5) Which of the following health care professionals carries out assessment of assaultive behavior risk factors?
A Clergy
B Environmentalists
C Nurse Aids
D Psychiatrists

6) The two identifiable types of assaultive behavior include
A Weapon-type and non weapon-type
B Inoculative and curative
C Associative and non associative
D None of the above

7) …..................... takes place when someone or a group of people attacks a person or persons using weapon or no weapon.
A Physical restrain
B Health Disorder
C Chemical restraint
D Physical assault

8) Physical assault may also take the form of rape
A True

B False

9) The Triggering phase is characterized by clear rage or agitation that is not easily concealed
A True
B False

10) A person with assaultive behavior cannot be arrested and placed under control by seeking help from mental health professionals.
A True
B False

11) Some possible causes of assaultive behavior based on clinical studies or history include the following, except
A Revenge
B Effective communication
C Anger
D Poor impulse control

12) Basically, ... stages of the assault cycle has been identified
A Five
B Three
C Eight
D Two

13) Which of the following phases is the outburst phase, in which the individual becomes totally uncontrollable?
A Recovery phase
B Escalation phase
C Crisis phase
D Triggering phase

14) Which of the following stages is the calming stage in which the individual's mood tends to be stable?

A Recovery phase

B Crisis phase

C Triggering phase

D Escalation phase

15) Internal factors that are linked with aggressive and violent acts include the following, except

A Humiliation

B Grief

C Sense of powerlessness

D Happiness

16) Which of these is not a physical factor that might cause violence?

A Heat

B Use of alcohol

C Balanced meal

D Lack of sleep

17) The use of medications to restrain the movement / behavior of aggressive people is called

A Chemical restraint

B Physical restraint

C Activity restriction

D None of the above

18) Medications used often as chemical restraint include the following, except

A Diazepam

B Epinephrine

C Haloperidol

D Lorazepam

19) Possible effects resulting from misuse or overuse of

drugs include the following, except
A Inability to feel pain
B Intact skin
C Choking
D Brain injury

20) Which of the following is not a characteristic of aggressive or violent patients
A. Aggressive people are capable of invading other people's spaces
B. Aggressive and violent patients communicate their aggression either verbally or non verbally
C Gestures in aggressive patients could be emphatic and usually appear as threat
D Aggressive patients tend to speak clearly and understandable

21) Some personal safety on the part of someone who might be become a victim of rage include the following, except
A Call a law enforcement agent such as police
B Avoiding direct confrontation with a violent-prone patient
C Walking towards the scene when you perceive imminent anger
D Walking away from the scene

22) Which of the following is a restraining technique used in aggressive behavior situations?
A Touch support
B Back head lock
C Front choke to the wall
D All of the above

23) In a psychiatric setting, restraining techniques

employed by nurses or other medical personnel include the following except

A Shouting at the violent patient

B Active listening skills

C The use of applicable verbal communication tactics to pacify violent and aggressive individuals

D How to use non-verbal communication skills to calm violent behavior

24) Strategies to avoid physical harm also involve simple self-defense techniques such as

A Wrist grabs

B Learning how to defend the face and the entire body

C Assuming a defensive standing posture

D All of the above

25) One of the effective techniques that experts employ in putting assaultive behaviors under control is

A to sue the patient to court for misbehaving

B To obtain patient history from a patient with assaultive or violent behavior

C To Create a harsh environment for the violent patient

D None of the above

The use of Restraint and Seclusion Review Questions

1. What does the acronym ISPN stand for

   A International Society of Psychiatric-Mental Health Nurses

   B Internal Society of Psychology- Mental Health Nurses

2. Registered nurses must not advocate for and protect the rights of patients

   A True
   B False

3. ISPN acknowledges that seclusion and restraint is an emergency clinical intervention employed as the first effort even though there is another restrictive alternative

   A True
   B False

4. Any physical method of restricting a patient's freedom of movement physical activity or normal access to his/her body is refer to as

   A Straight jacket
   B Choking
   C Restraint

5. In behavioral healthcare units, advanced practice _____ nurses are the best-qualified professionals to make assessments and decisions to restrain

   A Acute
   B Psychiatric
   C Neonatal

6. Who recommend that all patients receive thorough and ongoing assessment of their presenting behavioral problems

   A ISPN
   B ESPN

7. It is not imperative that providers concurrently screen and assess for co-morbid illnesses

   A True
   B False

8. Flexibility is adapting the environment of care is _____ to ensure safe and effective care for the least amount of time necessary to help patient regain control

   A Not effective
   B Not necessary
   C Mandatory

9. ISPN does not recommend that all staff members have specialize training in behavior assessment age-appropriate medication and safe monitoring

   A True
   B False

10. Physicians or licensed independent practitioner must perform a face-to-face assessments within _____ Hour of initiation of restraint

    A Half
    B 2
    C 1

11. The maximum a restraint can be in place for an adult is

    A < 4 hours
    B < 6 hours
    C < 8 hours

12. The maximum a restraint can be in place for adolescents ages 9-17 is

    A > 2 hours
    B < 2 hours
    C > 4 hours

13. The maximum a restraint can be in place for children 9 years old is

    A < 1 hour
    B < 4 hours
    C < 2 hours

14. Who does ISPN believes is best qualified to perform reassessments of restraints

    A CNAs
    B LVNs
    C Registered nurses

15. Children can be left alone while in restraint or while secluded

    A True
    B False

16. Adults and children must be removed from restraints every _____ hours at minimum

    A 1
    B 2
    C 3

17. Any medication administered to children must be ordered by physician or advanced practice nurse with prescriptive privileges

    A True

B False

18. _____ must be informed within 1 hour of the initiation of a restraint

A LVNs
B RNs
C Physicians or LIPs

19. ISPN does not recommend that the patient family members or significant others be informed immediately about the use of restraint or seclusion and receive written information

A True
B False

20. Family member should be included in patients' plan of care

A True
B False

Crisis Prevention and Intervention in Healthcare
Answers chapter 1

1. C
2. A
3. B
4. A
5. B
6. A
7. True
8. C
9. False
10. C
11. A
12. D
13. B
14. False
15. C
16. true
17. A
18. C
19. True
20. B

Crisis Prevention and Intervention in Healthcare
Answers chapter 2

1. D

2. A
3. B
4. C
5. D
6. B
7. A
8. C
9. A
10. B
11. A
12. D
13. A
14. A
15. True
16. False
17. True
18. True
19. True
20. True

Crisis Prevention and Intervention in Healthcare
Answers chapter 3

1. True
2. D
3. True
4. False
5. True
6. B
7. True
8. D
9. C
10. A

11. False
12. True
13. False
14. True
15. True
16. True
17. B
18. False
19. True
20. true

Crisis Prevention and Intervention in Healthcare
Answers Chapter 4

1. True
2. False
3. True
4. False
5. True
6. False
7. True
8. True
9. True
10. True
11. False
12. True
13. True
14. True
15. True
16. True
17. True
18. False
19. True
20. true

Crisis Prevention and Intervention in Healthcare
Answers Chapter 5

1. True
2. True
3. False
4. True
5. True
6. False
7. True
8. True
9. False
10. True
11. True
12. False
13. False
14. True
15. True
16. True
17. False
18. True
19. True
20. False

Crisis Prevention and Intervention in Healthcare
Answers Chapter 6

1. True
2. False
3. False
4. True
5. False
6. True

7. False
8. True
9. True
10. False
11. False
12. True
13. True
14. True
15. C
16. A
17. B
18. A
19. C
20. False

Crisis Prevention and Intervention in Healthcare
Answers Chapter 7
1. True
2. True
3. False
4. A
5. C
6. False
7. B
8. D
9. True
10. True
11. True
12. False
13. A
14. C
15. B

16. A
17. C
18. False
19. D
20. B

Answers to the Miscellaneous Review Questions

1. B
2. A
3. A
4. B
5. D
6. A
7. D
8. A
9. B
10. B
11. B
12. A
13. C
14. A
15. D
16. C
17. A
18. B
19. B
20. D
21. C
22. D
23. A
24. D
25. D

The Use of Restraint and Seclusion Answers

1. A
2. B
3. B
4. C
5. B
6. A
7. B
8. C
9. B
10. C
11. A
12. B
13. A
14. C
15. B
16. B
17. A
18. C
19. B
20. A

OTHER TITLES FROM THE SAME AUTHOR:

1. Director of Staff Development: The Nurse Educator (2nd Edition)
2. CNA Exam Prep: Nurse Assistant Practice Test Questions. Vol. One (2nd Edition)
3. CNA Exam Prep: Nurse Assistant Practice Test Questions. Vol. Two (2nd Edition)
4. IV Therapy & Blood Withdrawal Review Questions
5. Medical Assistant Test Preparation
6. EKG Test Prep
7. Phlebotomy Test Prep
8. The Home Health Aide Textbook (2nd Edition)
9. How to make a million in nursing 2015
10. Personality Types
11. How to Become a Better Wife
12. How to Become a Better Husband
13. How to Grow Your Small Business
14. It's in Your Hands: 5 Strategies to Achieving Your Life Dreams (Best Seller)
15. Weight Loss Inspiration

**Simply search "Jane John-Nwankwo"
on Amazon!**

**www.djngbooks.org
www.janejohn-nwankwo.com**

OTHER TITLES FROM THE SAME AUTHOR:

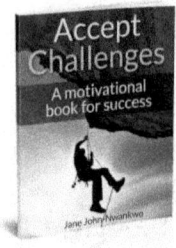
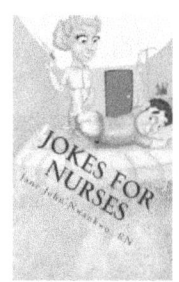
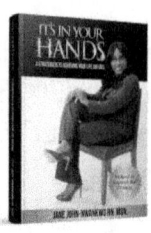

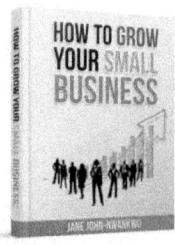
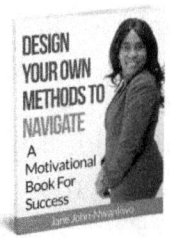
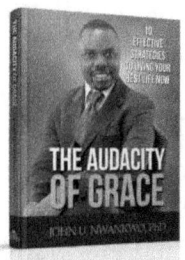

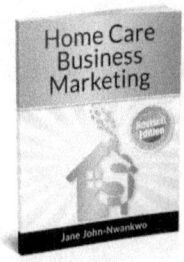
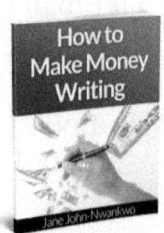
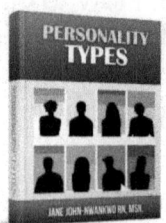

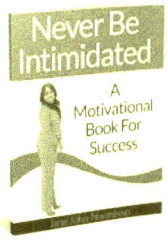

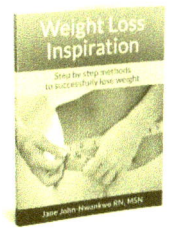

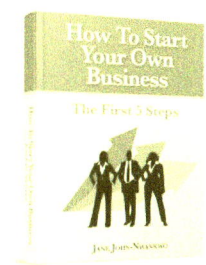

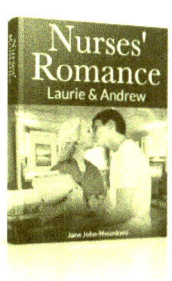

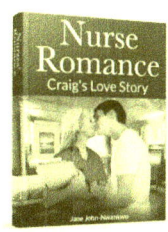

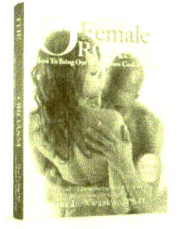

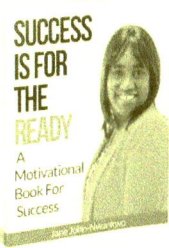

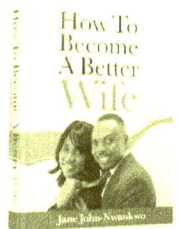

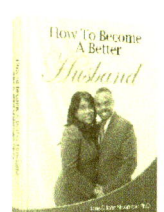

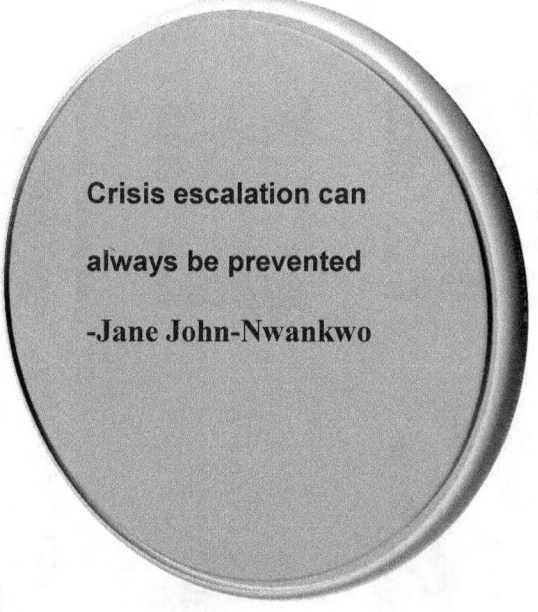

Crisis escalation can

always be prevented

-Jane John-Nwankwo

ABOUT THE AUTHOR

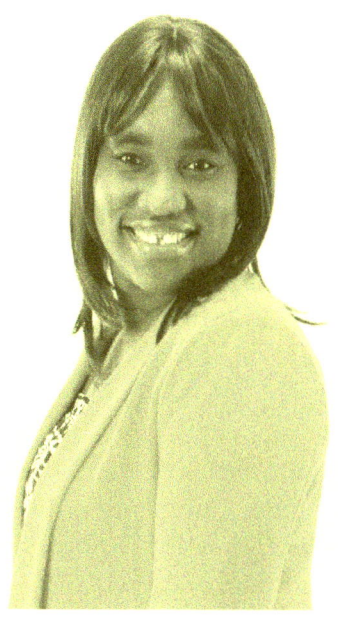

Jane John-Nwankwo CPT, RN, MSN, PHN is a motivational speaker and published author of more than 50 books which include textbooks for healthcare training, fiction for entertainment, and motivational books.
Simply search
"Books by Jane John-Nwankwo"
On Amazon.com

Visit her website:
www.janejohn-nwankwo.com

Book Jane John-Nwankwo as your motivational speaker now at www.JaneJohn-Nwankwo.com

With more than 10 years as a professional speaker, Jane John-Nwankwo can hold any audience sitting straight on their chairs for any length of time! She is a seminar leader and a published author of more than 50 books including textbooks for healthcare training, fiction for entertainment, books for new entrepreneurs and motivational and inspirational books like the "It's in your hands" series.

She received her Masters of Science in Nursing from University of Phoenix, and is currently pursuing a PhD in Nursing Science from University of Phoenix. Her speaking interests include: Motivational speeches for new business owners, Motivational speeches for any category of people, Employee seminars, Students' Empowerment, Healthcare topics, Topics related to women and any Christian topic. Book a speaking appointment today Wow! your audience. Electrify your seminar!!